Protocols for
MULTISLICE HELICAL COMPUTED TOMOGRAPHY
The fundamentals

Peter Dawson PhD FInstP FRCP FRCR

Department of Imaging
UCL Hospitals, London, UK

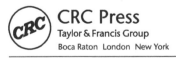

CRC Press
Taylor & Francis Group
Boca Raton London New York

CRC Press is an imprint of the
Taylor & Francis Group, an **informa** business
A TAYLOR & FRANCIS BOOK

CRC Press
Taylor & Francis Group
6000 Broken Sound Parkway NW, Suite 300
Boca Raton, FL 33487-2742

First issued in paperback 2019

© 2006 by Taylor & Francis Group, LLC
CRC Press is an imprint of Taylor & Francis Group, an Informa business

No claim to original U.S. Government works

ISBN-13: 978-1-84184-422-0 (hbk)
ISBN-13: 978-0-367-39120-1 (pbk)

British Library Cataloguing in Publication Data

Data available on application

Library of Congress Cataloging-in-Publication Data

Data available on application

Composition by Parthenon Publishing

Visit the Taylor & Francis Web site at
http://www.taylorandfrancis.com

and the CRC Press Web site at
http://www.crcpress.com

Contents

CONTENTS

Preface

The irreversible decline of computed tomography (CT) was predicted in the mid-1970s, as understandable excitement about the capabilities and potential of magnetic resonance imaging (MRI) burgeoned. However, with the development of 'spiral'/'helical' or 'volume scanning' technology, CT has confounded its detractors and has remained the imaging modality of choice for the resolution of many diagnostic questions, particularly in the chest and abdomen. Furthermore, entirely new applications such as CT angiography (CTA), high-resolution CT (HRCT) of the lung and virtual endoscopy and bronchoscopy have emerged and blossomed. The most recent technological development of all, the 'multislice' (up to 64) variant of helical CT, has cemented this renaissance by offering even higher speeds of acquisition, which allow either coverage of large body volumes in short times during a single breath-hold or coverage of more modest volumes at high and close to isotropic spatial resolution. The volume data sets thus obtained are ideal for multiplanar reconstructions and for such applications as virtual endoscopy and bronchoscopy. The zenith of this technology is represented by the 64-slice machines about to be delivered at the time of writing.

The design of image acquisition protocols without contrast enhancement offers little difficulty. Very little experience of CT is required to design an approach to covering a segment of, say, the abdomen with a chosen z-axis resolution in a time reasonable for a single breath-hold, whether single-slice or multislice technology is being used. The challenge becomes somewhat greater when an intravenous contrast agent is given, and attention has to be paid to the question of what contrast agent administration regimen is to be used, and to acquiring the scan at a time of optimal enhancement or if there is a need to obtain, say, two or more image acquisitions during different defined enhancement phases. In the past, with slow CT technology, the operator had little freedom in the design of contrast administration regimens, image acquisition protocols or the relationship of one to the other. Now, with a much faster pace of image acquisition, these matters have become critical, and poor choices may result in poor scans. A clear understanding of the fundamentals, particularly of contrast enhancement, will facilitate the rational planning of examinations.

It is for these reasons that special attention is paid in this small book to the subject of contrast agent pharmacokinetics. The purpose is to provide a simple introduction to the essential ideas involved, and a practical guide to implementation of rational protocols for the multislice spiral instruments based on them. The beginner may implement the protocols given uncritically, and may expect good results. In time, and with growing experience and confidence, he may develop his own, perhaps better, protocols. There is more than one pathway to grace, and to be too rigidly prescriptive would remove the art from medical imaging.

Peter Dawson
London

Introduction

This book, aimed primarily at radiologists and radiographers, has no pretensions to being much more than a collection of 'recipes', and simple ones at that, for contrast agent administration and computed tomography (CT) imaging. Recipe books may be very useful but, as any cook knows, there is rarely a 'correct' recipe for anything – although there certainly may be incorrect ones. It is much the same for CT. All the recipes promulgated here are for guidance only. Some experienced CT radiologists might do things quite differently and, they might argue, better. After some experience, the novice will undoubtedly want to be a little adventurous and add a dash of extra something or other to the recipes that he has initially rehearsed from the book.

The principal way in which the book departs from precedent in this area is in its first section, which seeks to present, in a largely non-technical, non-mathematical way, the pharmacokinetic basis of intravascular contrast agent enhancement. Few radiologists and radiographers have a clear grasp of this subject, and it is hoped that even those experienced in CT might also gain from reading it. Certainly, it seems to the author that some knowledge of this field should be an essential prerequisite for those intending to develop their own protocol variants.

The recipes given here are designed specifically for '64-slice' machines for two reasons. First, these machines will rapidly become the norm in our departments, and second, such fast machines present a challenge to those brought up, so to speak, on the slower incremental or single-slice spiral scanners, to modify somewhat regimens and protocols designed for a more leisurely pace of scanning. Failing to do so might, for example, lead to a situation in which an acquisition has been completed before the injection of contrast agent has ended, or, less dramatic but perhaps just as important, poor timing with respect to contrast administration of the start of a rapid data acquisition sequence may result in no part of the scan being obtained at a good time for contrast enhancement.

The two principal issues are:

(1) How much contrast agent of what concentration should be infused at what speed?

(2) When, with respect to the beginning and end of that infusion, should image acquisition be performed?

Another important question is: can less contrast agent be used with faster machines?

Although for the reason given above the regimens and protocols in the second part of this book have been laid down for 64-slice machines, an understanding of the basis of their design set out in the first part of the book will allow them also to be used for 4-, 8- and 16-slice machines, as will be explained later. Furthermore, notwithstanding their importance, little attention is paid in the book to a number of parameters. These include kV and mAs settings, kernels and filters. The reason for this is that it is difficult to prescribe these in a manner applicable to machines from all manufacturers, and it is therefore perhaps best to follow the manufacturer's advice on such matters, at least initially. Similarly, no space is devoted to suggestions on selection of images for hard-copy printing for either storage or reporting. PACS systems are with us more and more, and there is no question that reporting should now be done using soft-copy images on a dedicated workstation or a PACS (picture archiving and communications system) terminal. The axial, sagittal and coronal slice multiplanar reconstructions (MPRs) at the very least should be used in soft copy reporting.

This whole area is one in which terms are misused or used interchangeably, so it may be worth making an initial clarification. Above and in what follows we call the whole recipe for the CT scan a 'protocol', and the recipe for the contrast agent injection/infusion alone a 'regimen'.

Section I:

Some basic principles

1

Helical/spiral CT

It would be inappropriate in a book written for the purposes that this has been to delve, to any great extent, into CT technology. We summarise here only a handful of technical points important to the understanding of what follows.

In helical/spiral technology, the table moves continuously during rotation of the gantry carrying the X-ray source and detector arrays (Figure 1a). The origin of the term 'helical'/'spiral' is quite clear. The technique does not lead to the acquisition of a collection of axial slice images which may, if required, be assembled to obtain a volume data set, but, rather, to the primary acquisition of a volume data set from the outset, from which, if required, not only axial but any other planar slice reconstructions may be made or other image analyses carried out. The beam collimation width, say 0.6, 1.25, 2.5, 5 or 10 mm, dictates the z-axis spatial resolution.

In the case of a single-slice spiral machine (Figure 1b), if the table moves one collimation width in one rotation, the pitch is said to be 1 : 1, e.g. 10 mm collimation, 10 mm table movement per rotation. If the table feed per gantry rotation is, say, 1.5 times the collimation width (Figure 1c), the pitch is said to be 1.5 : 1, e.g. 10 mm collimation, 15 mm table feed per rotation. A greater pitch obviously reduces the image acquisition time for any physical length of scan (and the radiation burden), but it will also somewhat reduce the image quality and spatial resolution in the reconstructions in the z-axis. However, the loss of spatial resolution for the 33% reduction in imaging time in moving from pitch 1 to pitch 1.5 is modest and usually acceptable. Pitch calculated in this way is defined as:

pitch = (table movement per rotation)/(collimation (slice thickness))

In the case of a multislice machine, the X-ray beam is also 'fanned' in the patient axis (z) direction so as to fall on more than one ring of detectors

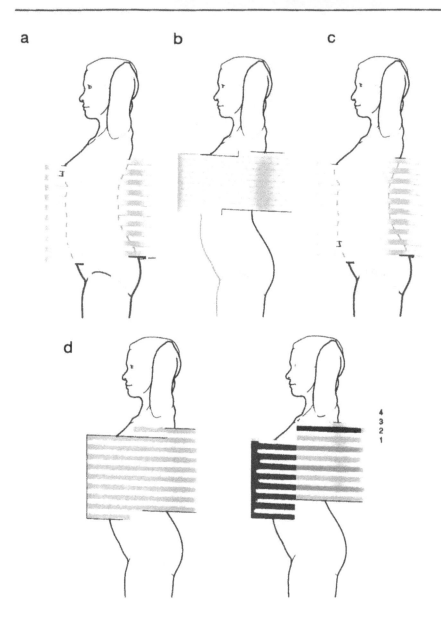

Figure 1   In (a) the origin of the terms 'helical' and 'spiral' are clear. In (b) and (c) the term 'pitch' is clarified by comparison of the two images: the first is pitch 1 (no overlap), the second pitch >1. With greater pitch the scans will be faster and the dose burden decreased. With pitch < 1 there will be overlap and, other things being equal, an increase in scan time and radiation dose. (a) and (d) illustrate single-slice, 2-slice and 4-slice spiral scanning

simultaneously (Figure 1d). Data acquisition at several times the rate achievable with a single slice machine is then possible, since a greater anatomical segment length may be covered per gantry rotation. For these systems another, more appropriate, definition of pitch is clearly necessary:

pitch factor = (table movement per rotation)/(*total* slice collimation)

This represents a more meaningful comparison with single-slice CT systems and is the definition adopted by the International Electrotechnical Commission (IEC). The pitch factor can be widely varied with the modern systems.

In multislice CT, the z-distance anatomical coverage per rotation is given by the product of the number of active detector slices and the collimation. The slice width actually obtained and available for reconstruction is the FWHM (full width at half maximum).

Once the essential input parameters and their possible combinations in a given manufacturer's system are understood, it is a straightforward matter to choose combinations of parameters. As an example, let us take an upper-abdominal segment of length 150 mm. The liver may be included, and suppose we want a high-resolution study of this, so then we may choose a 64×0.6 mm slice selection. If we have a 0.375 s gantry rotation time and a pitch of 1, the time of the acquisition will be:

$$[150/(64 \times 0.6)] \times 0.375 \text{ s} = 1.47 \text{ s}$$

The table speed will be:

$$150/1.47 = 102.4 \text{ mm/s}$$

Actually, there is no need to perform these calculations as the machine will indicate this result, but it is useful to have a grasp of the underlying ideas.

This is straightforward and can be quickly grasped. However, the above examples relate to a scan without contrast enhancement. If a contrast agent is given, as it usually will be for a liver study, it is obvious that the contrast injection regimen and the study protocol must be tailored one to the other. Furthermore, it is more usual that the liver will be only one part of the study, albeit an important one, and a study of the whole abdomen and perhaps other regions will more frequently be required. This makes matters a little more difficult, and showing how to set up the study so as to optimise timing in a variety of such circumstances is the aim of this book.

The combination of a little theoretical understanding of the importance of the principal parameters in spiral CT and the basics of descriptive contrast agent pharmacokinetics should give the reader confidence eventually to depart from any rigid prescriptions developed in this book and to design his own regimens and protocols for each situation on a rational basis.

Note that spiral technology may also be used in incremental (axial slice-by-slice) mode, with table movement only between single fixed-level slice acquisitions. Such incremental scanning *may* still have an occasional place in, for example, high-resolution lung studies and brain imaging.

TYPES OF IMAGE ACQUISITION

Multislice spiral/helical scanners may be used in a variety of modes as circumstances require. These include:

(1) The acquisition of large volume data sets, perhaps even of the whole body in trauma, at moderately high resolution in short times;

(2) The acquisition of more modest volume data sets at high isotropic resolution that are ideal for three-dimensional manipulations;

(3) The exploitation of shorter imaging times to obtain repeat image acquisitions of the same region in different phases of contrast enhancement, for example hepatic arterial and portal venous phases of the liver;

(4) Performing of single-level serial scans, where serial images at a single level, or at several levels simultaneously, allow the time evolution of contrast enhancement in a region of interest (ROI) to be recorded quantitatively as background subtracted CT numbers. From CT number versus time curves, perfusion, vascular volumes, capillary permeability and renal function may all be derived.

2

Contrast enhancement

X-ray contrast-enhancing agents are used to opacify the bowel and the arteries and veins and the organs they supply. The former are given orally and/or rectally; the latter are usually given intravenously, but, in some special applications, may be administered via an angiographic catheter into, for example, the superior mesenteric artery, the splenic artery or the hepatic artery (see below). The intravascular agents used in routine clinical practice are always iodinated, water-soluble X-ray contrast agents (ionic or non-ionic). It is assumed that it is almost universal practice to use non-ionic agents, as these are associated with a lower incidence of significant side-effects, such as vomiting, which might interrupt the scan, and because they are safer. No consideration will be given in this book to any specialist agents of other kinds.

The use of a contrast-enhancing agent is usually intended to achieve one or other of two objectives, or both: to 'label' bowel or blood vessels in order to identify them and to assist in distinguishing normal structures from abnormal (Figures 2 and 3); and to enhance the image contrast difference between a lesion and the normal background tissue in which it arises (Figure 4). It should be noted that success in neither aim is guaranteed. For example, it is not in the nature of the bowel that orally administered contrast should distribute itself uniformly throughout the whole length of the small and large bowel; nor is there any guarantee that lesions will be more conspicuous after intravascular contrast agent administration than before. In the liver, for example, a lesion may certainly disappear at one or more stages in the evolution of liver and lesion contrast uptake (Figure 5). Other generally less important reasons for intravenous contrast agent use include characterization of a lesion on the basis of its enhancement characteristics (of limited value for just a few lesion types), and for functional or physiological imaging (Figure 6).

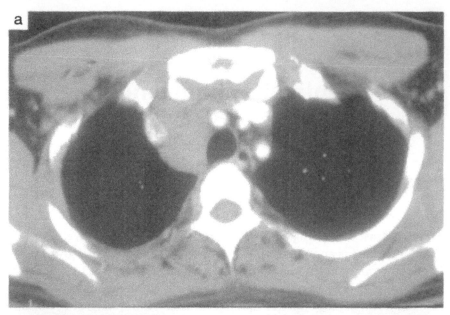

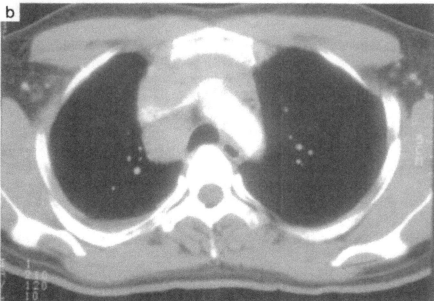

Figure 2 Blood vessels are 'labeled' with contrast agent and are thereby rendered easy to differentiate from other soft tissues. In (a) and (b) blood vessels are defined within the mediastinal mass; in (c) and (d) hepatic veins are identified following contrast agent and there is no possibility of their misinterpretation as lesions. The conspicuity of the lesion in the right lobe of the liver is also increased, rendering it clearly visible. Its dense peripheral nodular enhancement suggests a hemangioma, one of the small number of lesion types which may be diagnosed from their enhancement characteristics

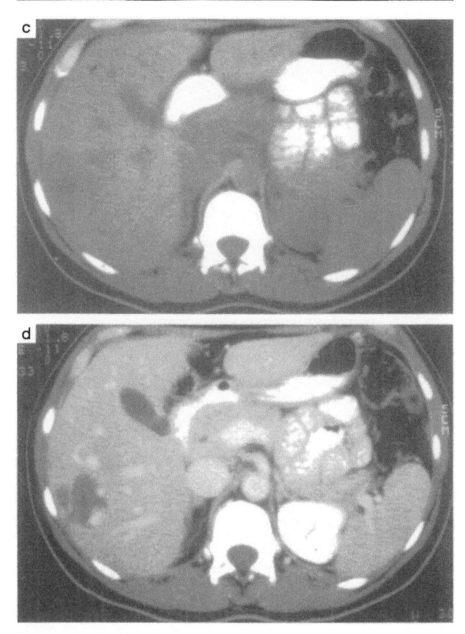

Figure 2 *(continued)*

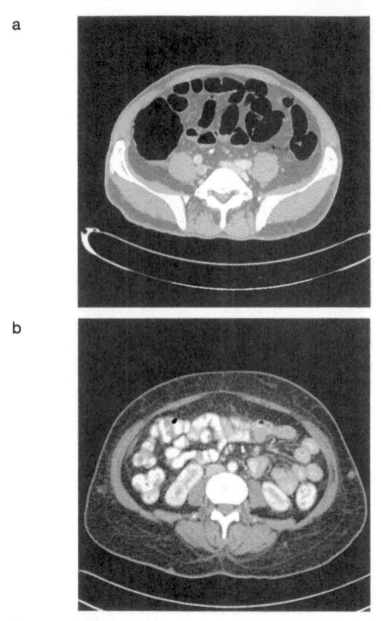

Figure 3 Bowel is 'labeled' with contrast agent and thereby rendered easy to differentiate from other soft tissues. In (a), (b) and (c) bowel is defined by negative (air), positive (barium in this case) and water contrast agent, respectively

It might be added that the use of a vaginal tampon in pelvic studies could be seen as another use of 'contrast' for labeling a structure. Here, gas in the interstices of the tampon material provides useful negative contrast.

c

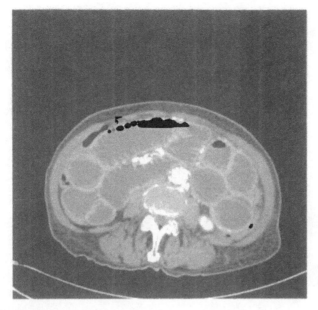

Figure 3 *(continued)*

BOWEL CONTRAST AGENTS

For abdominal studies, it is desirable to delineate the bowel from other structures such as lymph nodes, abdominal masses or abscesses. 'Positive' or 'negative' agents may be used.

Positive contrast agents used are either barium suspensions or iodinated agents. Different advantages and disadvantages are adduced for them. The behavior of barium suspensions is pH-dependent, and the pH varies through the gastrointestinal tract. Flocculation may occur and obscure lesions. Water-soluble iodinated agents are more commonly used. They have some peristaltic effect, and this tends to lead to a more homogeneous coating property. Furthermore, unlike barium suspensions, iodinated X-ray contrast agent solutions are safe if there is bowel pathology or perforation. On the other hand, in the presence of inflammatory bowel disease (which may be occult), there is a risk of absorption into the circulation and adverse reaction. If the solutions are made too dense, streak artifacts may degrade the image, and hence considerably diluted solutions are used. In the case of iodinated agents, these may be prepared by *ad hoc* dilution of a commercial intravascular preparation or of a commercial preparation designed for the purpose, the best known of which is Gastrografin (Schering AG, Berlin). Dilution to something of the order of 2% is usual.

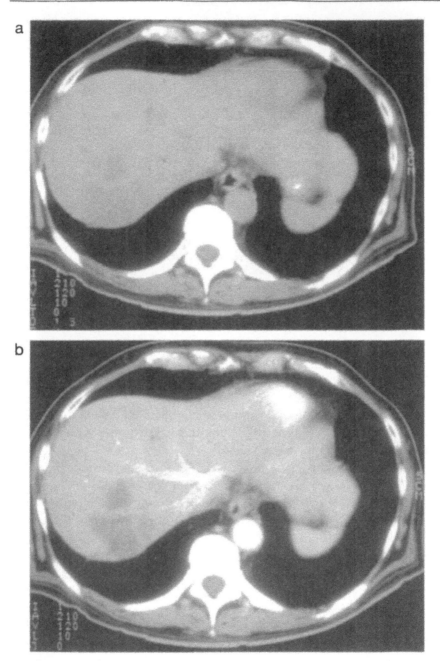

Figure 4 Increase in conspicuity of lesions following intravascular contrast administration. (a), (b) Demonstrate a low-attenuation lesion rendered readily visible as normal liver enhances to a greater extent than the lesion. (The same is seen in Figure 2c and d). In (c) a vascular lesion announces itself as a *higher*-than-background liver computed tomography (CT) number in the hepatic arterial phase

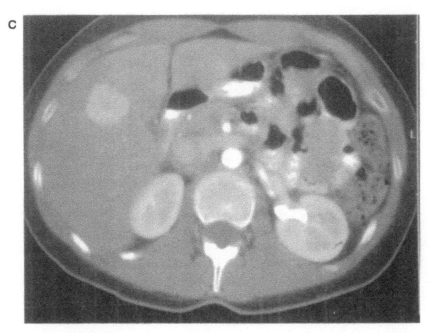

Figure 4 *(continued)*

Some radiologists give metoclopromide 20 mg with the oral preparation to speed gastric emptying and to achieve earlier bowel coating.

Barium preparations (e.g. E-Z-Cat®) are preferred by many, and are also given in dilute form, for example 1–2% concentrations.

Water alone, as a negative contrast agent, is an excellent alternative favored by many. In general, for abdominal studies such as liver, gall bladder, pancreas, gastrointestinal studies, focal lesion of the kidneys and CT angiography (CTA) studies, it is sufficient and perhaps preferable to use just water. Water is more effective than positive oral contrast agent in depicting the lining of the stomach and bowel in post-enhancement studies. In addition, the use of water will not obscure the blood vessels, thus allowing CTA processing to be performed easily afterwards.

For patients with suspected bowel perforation, only water or water-soluble contrast agent can be used. Barium suspension is contraindicated.

Timing of the oral administration of a contrast agent is important to ensure as even a distribution in the bowel as possible. Some guidelines are as follows.

Upper abdomen

A volume of 300 ml contrast agent diluted solution in three doses is recommended:

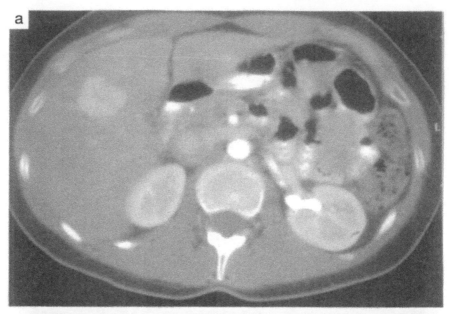

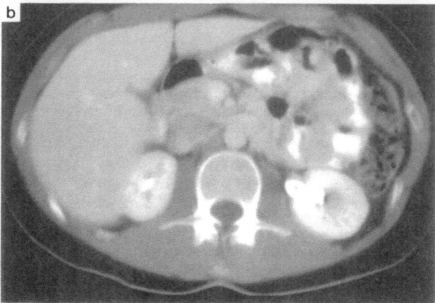

Figure 5 Conspicuity of a lesion does not necessarily increase following contrast administration, certainly not at all phases. Figures (a)–(e) illustrate lesions disappearing in different phases of scanning. In (a) a vascular lesion is seen in the arterial phase but disappears in a later phase (b). In (c), (d) and (e) a lesion barely visible in the precontrast phase (c) is seen clearly in the arterial phase (d) but disappears again in a later phase

c

d

e

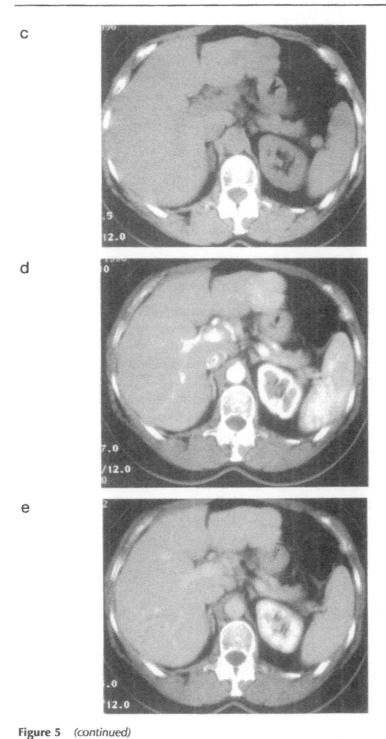

Figure 5 *(continued)*

First cup drunk 30 min before the study;

Second cup drunk 15 min before the study;

Thirrd cup drunk 5 min before the study.

To ensure adequate filling of the duodenal loop, some suggest laying the patient on the right side for 5 min before performing the topogram.

Abdomen–pelvis

A minimum of 800 ml of contrast agent diluted solution divided into four cups is recommended:

First cup to be drunk 1 h before examination;

Second–fourth cups every subsequent 15 min;

Start examination 5 min after the fourth cup is administered.

For pelvic studies, the first dose may be given 4–6 h before the examination, but, even so, one cannot assume that orally administered contrast agents will have reached the distal bowel by the time of the examination, so it is sometimes useful to administer rectal contrast agent in the same dilution as was given orally.

Rectal contrast agents may be required to delineate the rectum and sigmoid colon if a lower pelvic mass or pathology is suspected. In some cases, air may be substituted for a positive contrast agent. A very effective alternative is simply the insufflation of the rectum with air as a 'negative' contrast agent (Figure 7).

As already indicated, the use of a vaginal tampon may be helpful in adult female patients with suspected pelvic pathology. It is the author's belief that, too frequently, insufficient effort is made to optimize examinations of the pelvis that remain potentially among the most difficult of all to interpret.

INTRAVASCULAR CONTRAST AGENT ADMINISTRATION

The agents used for this purpose are all iodinated benzene-ring structures, and may be ionic or non-ionic, monomeric or dimeric. The chemistry, pharmacology, toxicology, tolerance and safety of these have been discussed extensively elsewhere. Here, we are interested only in an outline of their pharmacokinetics, since this dictates how they modify or 'enhance' the image and how this effect varies with time. It may be helpful first to comment on the widespread use of the word 'enhancement'.

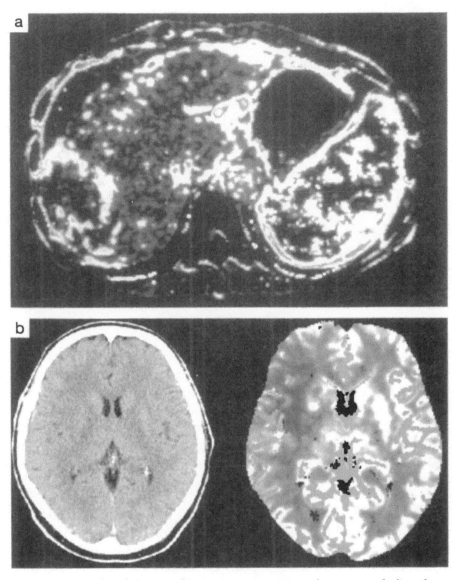

Figure 6 Examples of 'functional images': a parametric perfusion map of a liver (from *Functional CT* by Dawson, Miles and Blomley, Martin Dunitz) (a) and anatomical and parametric maps of the brain (b)

'Enhancement' of an examination is taken to mean simply the administration of an intravascular contrast agent. If, say, the liver is brighter, of higher CT number than baseline, then we usually say it is 'enhanced'. However, strictly speaking, what we seek to achieve by administering a contrast agent is an increase in the *difference* in CT number between one

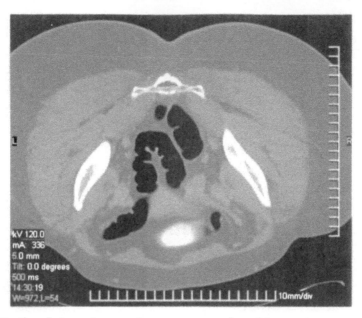

Figure 7   Rectal air used as negative contrast agent in pelvic scanning

region and another, between abnormal and normal, for example. That is to say, we seek usually to enhance the conspicuity of any lesion or to differentiate one structure from another. It should be understood that, as indicated earlier, there is no certainty that 'enhancing' the scan in the loose sense of the word will lead to enhancement of conspicuity of the lesion suspected, or sought. Indeed, a lesion may actually become less conspicuous as a result of 'enhancing' the scan, as already illustrated in Figure 5.

We will summarize the essentials of the pharmacokinetics of intravascular contrast agents in an almost entirely descriptive and non-technical manner. Although, at the margins, there are some slight differences in behavior between monomers and dimers and between ionic and non-ionic agents, these differences are small and clinically unimportant, and so will be ignored here. The description of the pharmacokinetics that follows may thus be considered valid for all current commercial intravascular agents. The choice of a specific agent type should be based only on questions of tolerance, organ-specific and systemic toxicities and the relative likelihood of significant associated idiosyncratic reactions, especially in at-risk patients. The non-ionic agents are of course superior in all these regards to the ionic agents. Following a general description of the pharmacokinetics, we will examine the special issues of faster versus slower injections, bolus injection versus infusion, the effects of concentration and total dose and the importance of different phases of enhancement, particularly in that important organ, the liver, with its dual blood supply. The crucial question is then considered as to whether protocols need to be adjusted as CT technology becomes faster: that is, can we use the same or must we use different protocols for multislice as opposed to earlier single-slice machines, for, say, 16-slice rather than 4-slice machines?

Pharmacokinetics of intravascular contrast agents

Pharmacokinetics is a specialist, technical subject with an essentially mathematical basis. However, we will present the necessary outlines of it here in a non-mathematical, descriptive manner, and illustrate the results of some such mathematical analyses pictorially. The reader who wishes to pursue this subject further is recommended to consult the references.

Iodinated X-ray contrast agents injected into the blood do not enter circulating cells but mix in the plasma. Because they are small molecules, they leak rapidly across normal capillary walls into the extravascular space, except in the brain where the intact blood–brain barrier (BBB) is impervious to the agents. Again, they do not significantly enter cells but distribute themselves in the extravascular, extracellular space (connective-tissue interstitium (IS)). This distribution between the plasma and interstitial spaces leads to a two-compartment pharmacokinetic model (Figure 8). During and immediately after injection, plasma/blood levels are high and IS levels are zero or low. The simple model assumes instant complete mixing of contrast agent with plasma. Then, as time goes on, IS levels rise because the contrast medium leaks into it, and blood levels fall because of this loss by leakage and, to a lesser extent, because of (slower) renal excretion. As is well known, this fall in plasma levels may be described by the sum of two exponential decays, one representing transfer to the IS, the other the renal excretion (Figure 9). A point comes when rising IS levels equal falling plasma levels and the curves cross (Figure 10). This is the 'equilibrium point', which will be discussed in some detail below. Thereafter, the IS concentration–time curve turns down and follows the plasma curve in parallel in the 'equilibrium phase'. There will now always be a slightly greater IS concentration than plasma concentration, and it is this which provides the gradient for clearing of IS contrast agent back into plasma for ultimate renal excretion.

In practice, the simple model is invalid, because mixing in the circulation is not instantaneous, and because, rather than using a rapid bolus

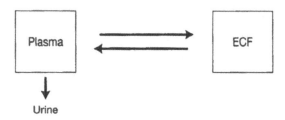

Figure 8 The two-compartment pharmacological model valid for water-soluble iodinated X-ray (and gadolinium chelate magnetic resonance imaging (MRI)) contrast agents. The first compartment is plasma (X-ray agents do not to any significant extent enter circulating cells) and the second is extravascular, extracellular space or 'interstitium' (again, the agents do not enter cells). ECF, extracellular fluid

injection, usually in CT we infuse contrast agent at a rate of, say, 3 ml/s. All the phenomena of mixing, leakage into the IS and renal excretion occur simultaneously. The blood/plasma levels do not become instantaneously high and then fall as in Figure 10. What is seen in practice is illustrated in Figure 11. The plasma (and blood) levels rise to a peak but at a decreasing rate, and thereafter fall, as shown, in a bi-exponential manner. Interstitial contrast agent concentrations rise and then fall much as before. Where the rising IS levels and the falling plasma levels cross in Figure 11b we have the 'equilibrium point'. Plasma concentrations have been plotted here (the factor linking plasma and blood concentrations is, of course, simply the hematocrit). Note, again, that the IS curve is not one that can in any practical way be observed. Note, too, that nothing is in any obvious equilibrium at the 'equilibrium point'. It is just that at that moment, since concentrations in the two compartments are equal, there is, instantaneously, no net transfer of contrast agent in either direction.

All this is a true description for any tissue in the body, but the specific curves in Figure 11b have been modeled for the liver. Notice how early the equilibrium point comes, at little more than 3 min or so after the commencement of infusion for this slow, 1 ml/s infusion, but depending somewhat on the infusion rate. This is important, since imaging of any tissue should be completed before the equilibrium point (see below). In practice, this is only an important fact to bear in mind when studying the liver, with its very early equilibrium point. In resting skeletal muscle, on the other hand, the equilibrium point comes very much later, at certainly more than 1 h.

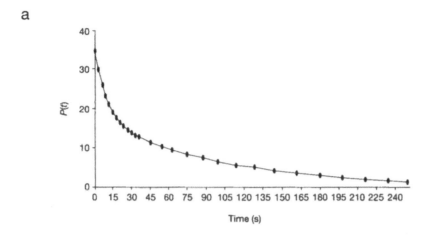

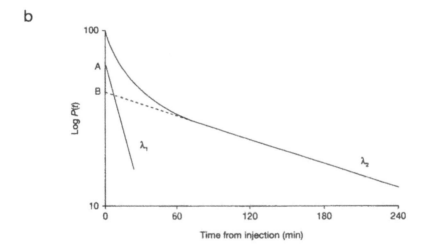

Figure 9 (a) Shows a modeled plasma (or blood) decay curve for intravascular contrast agent. The curve is bi-exponential with two decay constants (λ_1, λ_2). The first, of greater magnitude, describes redistribution between compartments (leakage to interstitium, effectively) and the second, of smaller magnitude, describes renal excretion. (b) Shows the result of expressing the concentrations as logarithms (semi-log plot): the later part of the curve becomes straight and its slope may be shown to be the glomerular filtration rate (GFR) per unit volume of extracellular fluid (ECF). $P(t)$, plasma concentration

The final step in this description is to consider what happens in a tissue region of interest (ROI). Consider the diagrammatic ROI of Figure 12. It makes the point that any such ROI contains both small blood vessels and IS, both of which contain concentrations of contrast agent varying

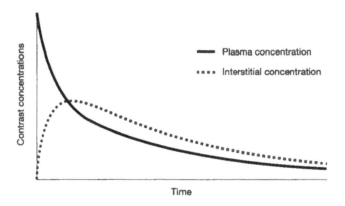

Figure 10 Declining plasma concentrations and increasing interstitial concentrations (diagrammatic). The curves cross at the 'equilibrium point' and thereafter decline in parallel throughout the 'equilibrium phase'

with time, as in Figure 11. It also contains cells, but these will have virtually no contrast medium in them. What is seen as a CT number for this ROI is a sum of IS and blood concentrations. It is, in fact, a weighted sum of these, because the contribution of blood contrast agent, for example, depends not only on the blood concentration but also on what proportion of the ROI is occupied by that blood. The situation is similar for the interstitial space. Using measured values for the fractional IS and blood volumes of tissue we can calculate the weighted sum. Figure 13 shows the result, again for the liver. Here blood, as opposed to plasma, concentrations have been plotted. We now have two curves that are observable in practice: the blood concentration curve from a blood vessel and the region of interest (ROI) curve. The position of the equilibrium point has been indicated on this diagram to illustrate the latest time by which a liver scan must be complete.

Varying infusion rates

Figure 14 shows the effect on blood concentrations of varying the infusion rate from 1 to 2 to 3 to 5 ml/s. Peaks come earlier and higher for faster rates, something that is intuitively reasonably obvious. Higher rates might therefore be considered to be better, especially for CT angiography. However, what is not so obvious is that the decline from the higher peak also occurs early, limiting the imaging window, and that the faster is the infusion, the earlier is the equilibrium point. The former is

a

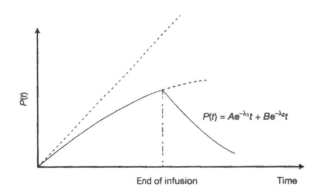

$$P(t) = Ae^{-\lambda_1 t} + Be^{-\lambda_2 t}$$

P(t)

End of infusion   Time

b

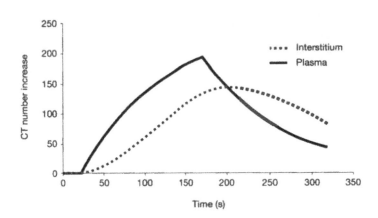

Figure 11 Figure 10, representing the standard pharmacological analysis for such two-compartment agents, assumes some initial plasma concentration in the circulation, ignoring how this is achieved. In imaging reality the usually ignored early phase of input of agent into the circulation is important. Diagrammatic (a) shows rising plasma levels (*P(t)*) as contrast agent is infused into the blood/plasma and levels rise. If all the blood vessels were impermeable there would be a linear rise of plasma concentration; because they are permeable the rate of rise steadily decreases, because the higher is the concentration in plasma the faster is the leakage to the interstitium. The curve tends toward an asymptote at which the concentration would be such that rate of infusion equals rate of leakage. In practice, of course, the infusion stops at some point and the bi-exponential decay described in Figures 9 and 10 is apparent. (b) Shows the result of mathematical modeling for the liver, both the plasma curve – in infusion (1 ml/s here) and decay phases – and the interstitial curve. The 'equilibrium point' is at their crossing point. *P(t)* is expressed here as CT number in (b)

a

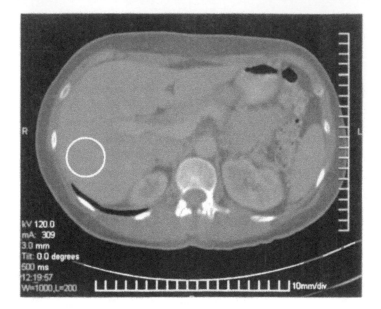

b

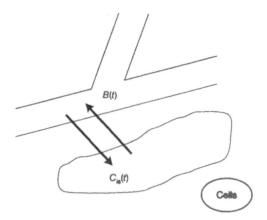

Figure 12 (a) A region of interest (ROI) drawn in the liver to avoid major blood vessels. (b) This ROI will contain microscopic vasculature, interstitium and cells. The first two will contain (time-varying) contrast agent concentrations, both of which will contribute to the CT number measured. In fact the net CT number (iodine concentration) will be a weighted sum of the two, the weighting factors being the fractional vascular ($B(t)$) and interstitial ($C_{is}(t)$) volumes in the ROI

apparent from Figure 14, and the latter is shown in Figure 15 in which IS curves are also plotted. If imaging must be completed before the equilibrium point, a later equilibrium point is desirable. A rate of 3 ml/s appears to be a good compromise in that reasonably high peak blood levels are

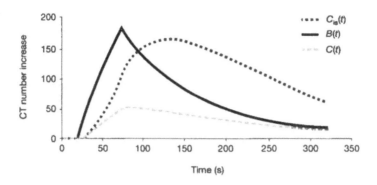

Figure 13 Modeled curves for the liver (blood ($B(t)$), interstitium ($C_{is}(t)$) and weighted sum ($C(t)$): ROI CT number). The blood and liver ROI curves are observable, unlike the interstitial curve, $C_{is}(t)$

achieved, and the equilibrium point is later than 2 min or so from the commencement of infusion. It may be seen immediately that to scan the whole liver at any reasonable z-axis resolution in the portal venous phase before the onset of equilibrium is almost impossible with an incremental scanner. However, with a spiral scanner, even single-slice, it is not a problem, as is discussed in more detail below.

Biphasic infusion regimens

Some authorities have suggested biphasic contrast agent infusion regimens, such as 5 ml/s for 10 s followed by 1 ml/s for 100 s. The idea is that high early levels might be achieved and then sustained by the slower infusion, while the equilibrium point will be delayed. Figure 16, comparing the results of a monophasic 3 ml/s injection with such a biphasic injection, confirms this theory. The equilibrium point is moved from 105 to 145 s. However, a more sophisticated contrast agent pump is required, and, as will be discussed below, this delay of the equilibrium point is not necessary if helical/spiral technology, either single- or multislice is available. Certainly, 64-slice machines make the concept totally obsolete.

The equilibrium point

There is considerable anecdotal evidence that examining an organ (usually the liver is the issue) in the 'equilibrium phase' may result in loss of conspicuity of some lesions. Theoretical considerations, which will not be reproduced here, also confirm that this should frequently be expected to be the case. It is important, therefore, to complete the study before this phase is reached, and, in the liver, this means completing it, as we have seen, before a little more than 2 min after the start of infusion. If we want to study the liver portal venous phase, we would not wish to begin acquisition much before, say, 70 s, when the ROI CT number is close to peak.

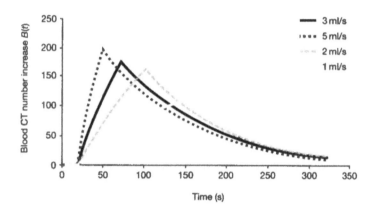

Figure 14 Blood concentrations ($B(t)$), expressed as CT number, achieved for different infusion rates

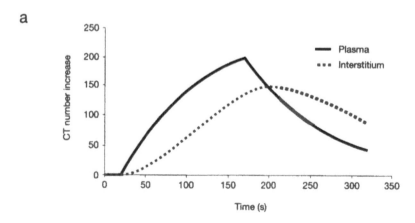

Figure 15 Plasma and interstitial curves (expressed as CT number) for different rates of contrast agent infusion illustrating the shifting position of the 'equilibrium point' for the liver: (a) 1 ml/s; (b) 2 ml/s; (c) 3 ml/s; (d) 5 ml/s. The faster the infusion the earlier the equilibrium point

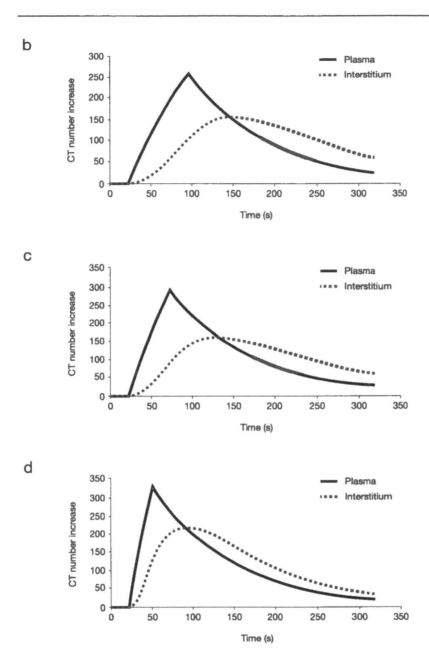

Figure 15 *(continued)*

This may give only about 50 s before the equilibrium phase begins. With spiral/helical imaging, this is easily long enough to scan a whole liver, even with narrow collimation and pitch 1. However, with incremental

a

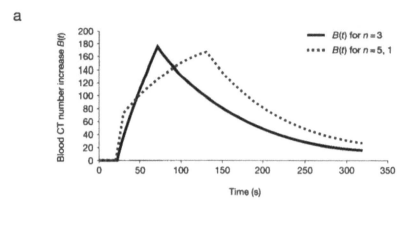

b

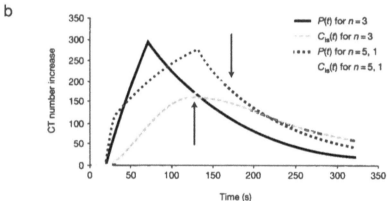

Figure 16 A biphasic (5 ml/s followed by 1 ml/s infusion) compared with monophasic infusion at 3 ml/s. The blood concentrations ($B(t)$) achieved are similar but somewhat more prolonged with the biphasic infusion (a). Additionally, when the plasma concentration ($P(t)$) curves are plotted and the interstitial curves are included, the biphasic infusion can be seen to delay the 'equilibrium point', albeit by a modest amount (b). $C_{is}(t)$, interstitial concentration

imaging, it is impossible to complete a typical liver study in 1 min. These facts are illustrated in Figure 17. Even if the study is begun a little earlier than is ideal, at, say, 50 s, the problem is not solved.

Modeling such as that described above, combined with clinical experience, permits the following summary of salient facts:

(1) Some factors are invariants to contrast agent injection regimen changes:

(a) The venous to arterial circulation time is a function of the patient and is not under the radiologist's control;

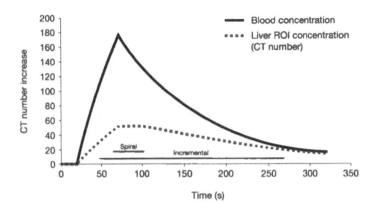

Figure 17 Modeled blood and ROI curves for the liver for an infusion rate of 3 ml/s of 300 mgI/ml contrast agent. The equilibrium point, not displayed here, we know from Figure 15 to be at approximately 130 s. Imaging must be complete by that time to avoid possible loss of lesion conspicuity. As can be seen, this is impossible with incremental scanning, but is not a problem with spiral/helical scanning

(b)   The time of arrival in the portal vein, similarly.

The cortico-medullary phase is 'immediate' (subject to point (a)), but the pyelogram is delayed some 3–5 min from intravascular injection.

(2)   The factors to be considered in enhanced CT are vascular enhancement (blood contrast agent concentrations) and tissue/organ ROI enhancement (a weighted sum of microvascular and interstitium contrast agent concentrations). In CT angiography the former alone is of interest; in any other examination the latter is of greater importance.

(3)   Intravascular contrast agents are sometimes helpful simply to 'label' blood vessels, to help in image interpretation in the same way that oral or rectal contrast agent may be used to label bowel. For this purpose, only modest levels of contrast agent are necessary, and precise timing is not critical.

(4)   For CT angiography (CTA) proper, higher blood levels maintained throughout the scan are, of course, required, and timing *is* critical. This will be discussed further below. Faster injections of the same total dose give higher peak blood flow values at earlier times, but the high values are sustained for a shorter period. This may be seen from Figure 15.

(5) The magnitude of arterial enhancement achieved is a function of contrast agent concentration, infusion rate and total time of infusion.

(6) Apart from CTA, the principal reason for intravascular contrast agent administration is to increase the contrast between structures, to render them more visible and, in particular, to enhance the difference between normal and abnormal tissue CT numbers, to increase lesion conspicuity. It has been shown, incidentally, both in clinical practice and theoretically, that the conspicuity of typical relatively hypovascular liver lesions increases as the normal liver tissue CT number increases. This suggests that not too great an emphasis on economy in contrast agent use would be the best policy.

(7) Varying infusion rates over the range typically used clinically have different effects on arteries and organs. The magnitude of arterial concentrations is proportional to the flux of agent, i.e. to (flow rate × concentration). Conversely, the portal venous phase enhancement of the liver is quite insensitive to changes in contrast agent administration flux over this range, but depends more simply on total load administered. The magnitude of organ, e.g. hepatic, enhancement is a function of total iodine dose administered, and may be adjusted by changes in concentration of agent administered, total volume or both.

On the other hand, where the hepatic arterial phase of liver enhancement is of interest, this *is* injection rate-dependent. Regarding faster injections, it is important to note that there is, in fact, little to be gained by pushing the infusion rate beyond about 5 ml/s, since the right heart and lungs represent a buffer, preventing achievement of higher and higher concentrations by faster and faster injections.

(8) Any tissue or organ must be examined in its entirety before the 'equilibrium phase', the time of onset of which is itself, to a significant degree, a function of infusion rate. This argument is valid for any organ but is critical for liver imaging, since equilibrium is established very early in the liver.

(9) Prior to the introduction of helical CT, injection rates were prolonged, and experiments with two-phase injections were done in an effort to delay the onset of equilibrium. Additionally, portal venous phase scanning was often started much too early in terms of contrast enhancement, in order to beat this deadline, so to speak. The

result was scans of the liver which were suboptimal in enhancement for the early slices, and probably, in spite of all efforts, actually nevertheless in the equilibrium phase for the later ones.

(10) The speed of the machine determines its ability to record image data during the most advantageous time period, e.g. maximized arterial enhancement, the pre-equilibrium phase in the liver or individual phases in true multiphasic imaging.

(11) Even though image acquisition may now be very fast, we cannot argue that as a consequence the imaging time window may now be allowed to be narrow. A narrow window may easily be missed. A reasonably wide time window for imaging remains desirable. The exploitation of bolus-timing software is essential.

(12) Cardiac output has a significant influence on timing of arrival and peak of contrast agent in the arteries (relevant to CTA). However, although there will be a delay in peak enhancement in the liver too, this will be little affected, except in extreme cases, since this is much more dependent on the total dose delivered.

(13) Interestingly, and counter-intuitively, a reduction in cardiac output will result in an increase in peak arterial enhancement. The fundamental explanation for this is that, with a lower cardiac output, less blood is ejected from the heart to dilute the contrast agent during transit, and in practice this overrides the effect of a prolonged transit time working in the direction of reducing peak enhancement. Of course, all this is true only up to a point – zero cardiac output will deliver no contrast agent at all to the arteries.

(14) For a given contrast agent load, arterial and organ enhancements are inversely proportional to body mass, so the contrast agent total load to body mass ratio is a key determinant of enhancement.

How much must data acquisition speed be taken into account?

The introduction of faster machines, be it multislice versus single-slice or 64-slice versus 4-slice, would seem to suggest that we might substantially modify contrast agent injection regimens advantageously in order to use less contrast agent, perhaps more rapidly injected, both in the interests of the patient and with financial gains. However, some of the fundamentals outlined above indicate that little in this regard can usefully be achieved. The following discussion of some general image acquisition principles with examples illustrates this.

CT ANGIOGRAPHY

This may be seen as a special case and perhaps the easiest to get right with bolus triggering. In all other CT examinations it is the combination of vascular and extravascular contrast agent that affects the enhancement; in the case of CT angiography it is, by definition, the intravascular agent concentration alone that contributes. Here we may state some basic principles:

(1) An adequate blood concentration of contrast agent must be achieved and sustained during the time of the data acquisition.

(2) Data acquisition during a single breath-hold (where a breath-hold is necessary) of around 20 s should be the aim.

(3) Accurate timing of the start of data acquisition should be achieved using bolus-timing techniques.

(4) On the basis of point (3), point (1) may be achieved by approximately matching contrast agent infusion time to necessary imaging time. This in turn may be seen to determine the total dose required.

It is more convenient in CTA to think in terms of flux of contrast agent, i.e. (rate of infusion × concentration). This may be increased to achieve higher blood concentrations, and consequent improved signal-to-noise ratio, by increasing the rate of injection, increasing the concentration of the contrast agent preparation or both. Some would argue that in this application a higher-concentration formulation of the agent is useful. As has been noted earlier, however, there is little to be gained by pushing the infusion rate beyond about 5 ml/s. The total dose to be delivered is then dictated by the desirability of approximately matching the infusion time to the scan time, as suggested above. One misunderstanding might helpfully be cleared up here. There is a widespread perception that prolonged infusion achieves a plateau of contrast agent concentration in blood vessels. This is not the case: concentrations continue to increase, albeit at an ever-slower rate, and become asymptotic to a plateau never reached (Figure 18).

The application and consequences of these principles will be illustrated by a few examples of CTA. Examples for 4- and 16-slice machines

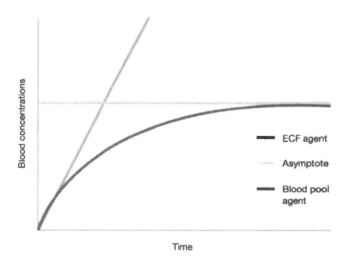

Figure 18 Blood concentration of a blood pool agent and of an extracellular fluid (ECF) agent. Plasma/blood concentrations approach an asymptotic value at which rate of infusion would equal rate of leakage to the interstitium

will be used to illustrate how marked might be the changes brought about later by 64-slice machines.

Aortoiliac CTA

Such a study might, for example, be done for suspected abdominal aortic aneurysm. The extent of the region of the abdominal aorta and the iliac vessels to the level of the proximal femoral vessels is some 40 cm. Using a 4-slice machine, 4×1.25 mm collimation, a pitch of 1.5 and a gantry rotation time of 0.5 s (dictating a table speed of 15 mm/s), this can be covered in about 25 s, perhaps just comfortable for an average breath-hold. If an infusion rate of 5 ml/s is chosen to obtain high levels of contrast agent, then about 125 ml of contrast agent would give a match of acquisition and infusion times.

Obviously, data acquisition should not begin until reasonable concentrations have been infused.

To study the smaller volume needed for renal artery assessment, say no more than 20 cm in extent, the acquisition time is approximately halved, so the total contrast agent dose required is halved. However, this in turn will have a consequent impact on contrast agent concentrations achieved, as discussed below under 'Very short acquisition times'.

Thoracolumbar aortography

This is an anatomical block of greater length, say some 60 cm, and were the above parameters to be used with a 4-slice machine the scan time would be 40 s (a not so easy breath-hold, although with a cephalocaudad scan breathing during the later pelvic portion would not be disastrous), and the 5 ml/s infusion rate would dictate a total dose of some 200 ml. This is unacceptable, and the choices would be: reducing the injection rate to, say, 3 ml/s, accepting a lower blood concentration and reducing the contrast agent load to 120 ml; accepting a reduced z-axis resolution by scanning at 4×2.5 mm collimation to halve the scan and infusion times; or using an 8- or 16-slice machine capable of covering the region at the same high z-axis resolution in a significantly shorter time.

Aortobifemoral CTA

The distance from the distal infrarenal abdominal aorta to the ankles is some 120 cm. With a 4-slice machine, 4×2.5 mm collimation, a pitch of 1.5 and a gantry rotation time of 0.5 s (dictating a table speed of 3 cm/s), this would be covered in about 40 s. With an infusion rate of 4 ml/s the infusion total load would be a rather large, 160 ml – and this for a not very high z-axis resolution. The answer here is clearly to use an 8- or 16-slice machine, since even dropping the infusion rate to 3 ml/s would be of little help in limiting the contrast agent dose if 4×1.25 mm acquisition was decided upon.

The essential point concerning total doses in CTA is not so much that they can be reduced with faster and faster machines (see 8-slice and 16-slice examples above), but, rather, that good CTA could not previously be achieved at all.

Very short acquisition times

There is an important point to be made about very short acquisition time scans taking less than, say, 20 s, and the need ideally to match scan and injection times. Two problems arise: first, timing becomes even more critical because of the narrow time window, and second, the contrast agent concentrations reached in blood after a short infusion time matched to a short data acquisition time will be relatively low. Regarding the latter problem, two strategies may be adopted. The contrast agent flux may be increased; this is achieved by the use of a higher-concentration formulation rather than by an increase in rate of injection, since the latter, as previously discussed, is of little help above about 5 ml/s; or, alternatively, a longer infusion may be carried out and the scanning commenced later when blood levels are higher. This last point is a crucial one with 64-slice machines, which may be thought of as 'ultrafast'. Thus, consider the aortobifemoral study example above, an anatomical length of some 120 cm as performed with a 64-slice machine with a rotation time of 0.375 s. If we select a high-resolution mode and utilize 64×0.6 mm collimation and a pitch of 1, the scan will be completed in:

$$[120 \times 10 \text{ mm}/(64 \times 0.6) \text{ mm}] \times 0.375 \text{ s} = 12 \text{ s}$$

At an infusion rate of 4 ml/s this would be less than 50 ml of contrast agent, rather a low dose even if a higher concentration were to be used. Even at 5 ml/s the volume would be only 60 ml.

The obvious recourse is to commence scanning at, say, 20 s, by which time 80 ml would already have been delivered (at 4 ml/s). The scan would be completed by 32 s so a total load of 128 ml would be used.

The question as to whether total contrast agent doses can be reduced with multislice CT is, as regards CTA, something of a non-question in that only now, with 16- to 64-slice machines, can the procedure be done well. In this sense there are not good before and after procedures to compare and the relative dose issue is secondary and meaningless. What can be said is that savings in contrast agent dose are not easy to make because certain minimum blood concentrations must be reached. If super-fast systems are used to reduce the scan time (as they have to be with larger anatomical volumes, as illustrated above in the aortobifemoral example), the injection time, which needs to be matched to it, is reduced. If the injection time is short, only low blood levels will be achieved unless the contrast agent flux during the short time period of injection is very high. Since injection rates higher than about 5 ml/s are not much more effective, the only options are to increase contrast agent concentration and/or to prolong the injection time to deliver more contrast agent, and to delay imaging until the higher levels have been achieved. As far as CTA is concerned, therefore, the scope for contrast agent savings with faster scanners would seem to be limited by fundamentals.

ABDOMINAL IMAGING

One may take a simple view and say that in virtually all abdominal imaging the liver will also be imaged and should be imaged optimally. On this assumption we conclude that the delivery of contrast agent has to be tailored to this end, with other organs being imaged, perhaps, earlier or later in the evolution of the distribution of contrast agent, as appropriate. Therefore, liver imaging will be considered first.

The liver

The issues surrounding the two blood supplies of the liver are well enough understood. We are most often interested in the portal venous phase. As discussed above, this does not occur maximally until some 60–70 s after commencement of infusion. Fast multislice systems allow the commencement of scanning in this phase to be delayed until some such time that, with confidence, the whole liver may be covered, even at highest z-axis resolution, before the onset of equilibrium.

Furthermore, it has been shown that the conspicuity of hypovascular liver lesions, the usual issue, increases as normal liver enhancement increases in the portal venous phase. Thus, leaving aside the question of timing, the enhancement of the liver via its principal blood supply is a function of the total dose given. It follows that it is unlikely that we can achieve more than a marginal reduction in total dose administered by using faster injections.

It is worth noting here that there is a divergence between mainstream and European practice, in that a typical European total dose for a liver study would be 120 ml of 300 mgI/ml concentration agent, whereas a typical US dose would be 150 ml.

Hepatic arterial phase imaging

In the context of a contrast agent administration regimen tailored to optimize liver portal venous phase enhancement, any other imaging can be incorporated; for example, the hepatic arterial phase of the liver, the cortical nephrogram phase of the kidneys and the arterial phase of the pancreas may be obtained in an early scan. Since an element of optimization of these is clearly appropriate, a higher injection rate of the agent may be used, say 4 or 5 ml/s rather than 3 ml/s.

The parenchymal phase of the pancreas may be obtained at, say, 35 s, and a portal venous phase sequence incorporated into the liver study will demonstrate a good parenchymogram but now with good demonstration of venous drainage also.

A 'delayed phase' of the kidneys, where required, may simply be obtained in a third scan.

In the more unusual circumstances that *only* the kidneys, pancreas or spleen, say, were to be imaged, then this could be achieved with a significantly smaller total dose of agent.

Thus, in summary, while it would seem that shorter infusion times of consequently lower total doses of contrast agent might be possible in CTA with faster machines, this ignores the fact that a shorter injection will only achieve lower blood concentrations. This cannot be effectively offset by faster injection rates, as rates greater than some 5 ml/s will achieve little, and will increase the risk of extravasation significantly. It may be offset to a limited extent by using higher-concentration formulations of contrast agent, but adequate levels will probably only be achieved by combining this with a prolongation of injection and a delay of commencement of the short scan sequence until higher blood levels are reached. Obviously, these maneuvers militate against achieving dose reductions. Similarly, regarding all other CT organ imaging, physiological and pharmacological fundamentals dictate that only a marginal reduction in the total dose of contrast agent may be achieved using faster infusions and exploiting the faster feeds of multislice CT. In short, there is no clear need, and little to be achieved, by modifying for faster systems the protocols developed for slower systems.

Technique of infusion

A cannula of sufficient caliber to accept a flow rate of at least 3 ml/s or so is chosen and placed in a suitable vein, usually antecubital. Multiple puncture attempts increase the risk of extravasation. It is desirable to stay with the patient for the first 10 s or so of the infusion to check for extravasation. A pump injector should always be used for reliability and reproducibility of infusion regimens. At least one modern injector has an extravasation detector system.

Bolus timing

Various bolus-timing software is built into commercial machines, such as 'Smart Prep' or 'CARE Bolus'. These are most useful when a poor cardiac output/prolonged circulation time is suspected.

Total iodine dose

Regarding this, it is difficult to be prescriptive. Account must be taken of patient body mass and smaller total doses given to children. Suggestions such as 'adults': '2 ml/kg body weight' are not entirely helpful, as agent concentration is not given. There is a difference in approach between Western Europe and the United States, smaller total doses being typically used in the former than in the latter. Thus, 100–120 ml of 300 mgI/ml concentration agent might be a European regimen, and 150 ml of 300 mgI/ml concentration agent a more typical US regimen. Thought must be given to renal function in CT studies using substantial volumes of intravascular contrast agent.

SPECIAL TECHNIQUES

Usually, contrast agent is infused intravascularly into a peripheral vein, but in the study of the liver some special approaches are occasionally used.

CT hepatic arteriography

This is now a rarely performed procedure. An angiographic catheter is inserted in the hepatic artery and the patient transferred to the CT suite. A rapid bolus injection is performed, and imaging commenced at about 10 s. This is close to the peak hepatic arterial contrast agent concentrations. Hypervascular lesions such as neuroendocrine, carcinoid and melanoma metastases will enhance more than the normal liver, since they are relatively vascular and their blood supply is primarily hepatic arterial, whereas that of normal liver is primarily portal venous (Figure 19a). The whole liver should be imaged before the portal venous contrast agent arrives. This is quite feasible with both single- and multislice spiral but not with incremental systems.

CT hepatic arterioportography (CT portography)

Here, an angiographic catheter is placed in either the splenic artery or, more typically, the superior mesenteric artery, and the patient is transferred to the CT suite. Contrast agent is injected into the artery and scanning commenced, say, 20–25 s later when the portal venous return peaks. Now, normal liver should exhibit strong enhancement, but any tumor, which receives its blood supply predominantly from the hepatic artery, does not enhance, and appears as a 'filling defect' in the liver (Figure 19b). A number of artifacts due to perfusion variations and deficits have been noted in such studies, which are capable of causing confusion and false-positive diagnoses.

Delayed CT

This term is used in quite different ways. First, it is used to describe a study done just a few minutes later than the routine studies in one or two circumstances, e.g.:

a

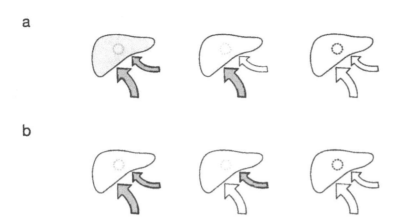

b

Figure 19 The liver has two blood supplies, hepatic arterial and portal venous. The normal liver is supplied predominantly by the latter, and tumors predominantly (but variably) by the former. This is the basis of understanding liver enhancement, liver embolization and special techniques such as CT hepatic arteriography (CTHA) and CT portography (or arterioportography, CTAP). In (a) CTHA is demonstrated. Direct infusion of contrast agent via a catheter placed in the hepatic artery will result initially in enhancement primarily of any tumor, with little enhancement of normal liver; later, when contrast agent arrives in the portal vein (in relatively diluted concentrations), the normal liver will be enhanced and will tend to catch up the lesion which may 'disappear'. In (b) CTAP is illustrated. Here, contrast agent is infused directly into the splenic artery or superior mesenteric artery and on venous return directly fills the portal vein, thereby strongly enhancing normal liver but not tumor, which tends to appear as a filling defect. Later, in the equilibrium phase, the lesion may 'disappear'

(1)   Suspected hemangioma: such lesions 'fill in' from the periphery over a period of a few minutes (Figure 20).

(2)   Suspected cholangiocarcinoma: these may exhibit 'retention' of contrast/persistent enhancement, as compared with normal liver, at about 5 min.

Second, the term is occasionally used to denote a much longer delay of 4–6 h. This technique was originally proposed on the following basis. Although, as indicated above, contrast agents do not significantly enter cells, about 1% of an administered load is in fact taken up into hepatocytes. This is not enough to make an impact on any of the pharmacokinetic arguments used above or to make any impact on routine scanning. However, at 4–6 h, this 1% or so is still retained in hepatocytes, whereas the concentration of contrast agent in blood and the IS is virtually zero. This is enough to give the normal liver a 20-HU (Hounsfield unit) or so residual enhancement above the precontrast administration baseline.

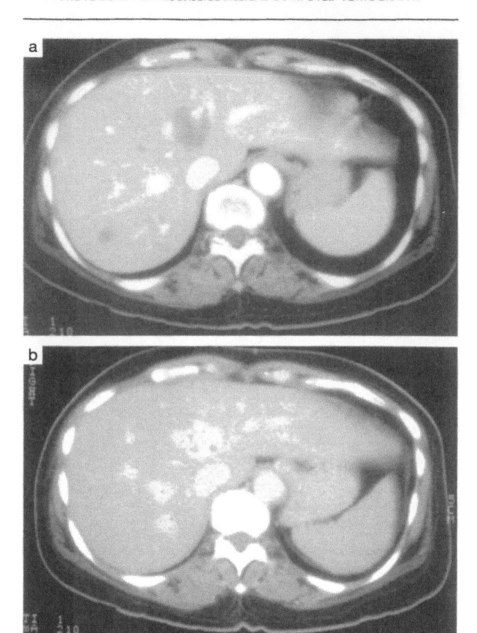

Figure 20 Early on, a hemangioma exhibits peripheral nodular enhancement (a), and tends on delayed scans to 'fill in', albeit frequently incompletely (b). A further characteristic, insufficiently emphasized, is that at any stage the enhancement seen parallels that in blood vessels

Liver tumors that do not contain normal hepatocytes do not exhibit this effect, and therefore appear as filling defects. This technique has not been widely used because of the inconvenience of recalling a patient for the delayed scan, but it has proved useful on occasion in resolving persisting uncertainty about artifacts versus real lesions in CT portography, for example.

Single-level serial images

Repeat images of a single slice or several slices simultaneously with a multislice system following contrast agent injection allows ROI CT number–time curves to be obtained (Figure 21). The initial rise in CT number clearly reflects blood flow, or, to be precise, perfusion. Simultaneous examination of a local blood vessel CT number–time curve allows an unraveling of the blood versus IS contributions to the ROI CT number at any instant. The rate of change of IS levels reflects capillary permeability. A mathematical analysis is necessary to take these ideas further quantitatively, and this will not be given here. Such analysis allows parameters including regional perfusion, vascular volume, interstitial volume, capillary permeability and glomerular filtration rate (GFR) to be derived from serial single-level CT data acquisitions. The reader is referred to the literature for further details.

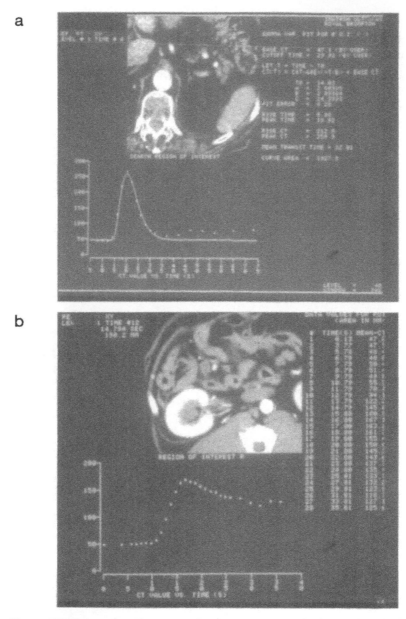

Figure 21　CT number–time curves for the aorta (a) and the kidney (b), which are the basis for functional studies

3

Patient preparation and drugs

Emergency imaging and imaging on very ill patients may be performed, of course, without any preparation. Indeed, multislice machines may be particularly useful, for example, in performing rapid, virtually whole-body, scans in (obviously unprepared) trauma patients.

In more routine scans a 'nil by mouth' regimen for at least 4 h or so is recommended if the patient is to receive an oral contrast agent or water, as the large volume which must be drunk would be difficult to tolerate on a full stomach. This is also recommended if an intravascular contrast agent is to be administered in case the patient should vomit, although this is unlikely with the non-ionic agents.

The nil by mouth prescription is best interpreted narrowly as meaning no solids or milk products. Clear fluids in modest volumes are perhaps to be encouraged, as dehydration should be avoided. Indeed, if the patient cannot drink clear fluids, a drip should be set up to avoid dehydration at the time of the contrast agent study, in the interests of protecting renal function.

Other than contrast agents given orally, rectally or intravascularly, few drugs are used in clinical CT. Metoclopromide has been recommended, but is little used, as an adjunct to oral contrast agents to encourage gastric emptying and contrast agent distribution of the agent through the bowel.

PREMEDICATION AND PROPHYLAXIS

Some authorities recommend the use of corticosteroid prophylaxis against major adverse reactions in patients with definable risk factors. A typical approved regimen would be oral prednisolone 40 mg twice, the day before the examination. However, it should be noted that the evidence for the efficacy of such a regimen is not clear-cut. Some authorities, alternatively, recommend prophylactic antihistamines in such patients. The author recommends simply the use of non-ionic agents without other disruptive drug regimens of unproven worth.

A number of approaches to the prophylaxis of contrast-associated nephrotoxicity have been proposed but none are of proven efficacy.

ALTERNATIVES TO IODINE

Gadolinium chelate contrast agents designed for use in magnetic resonance imaging (MRI) have been recommended for use in CT in patients at high risk for adverse reaction to iodinated agents. However, high doses outside the range approved are necessary to achieve good results, and they are expensive. The idea that they are also associated with reduced renal effects is probably untrue at the higher doses.

SEDATION AND ANESTHESIA

Patients who are anesthetized or heavily sedated should, of course, be attended in the scanner suite by an anesthetist or other appropriately qualified person. Satisfactory monitoring cannot be achieved from the control console several meters away. This monitoring difficulty in patients in general has, in fact, been cited as an indication for using safer non-ionic agents exclusively in CT scanning.

In the anesthetized, intubated patient, suspension of respiration for brief periods may be organized with the assistance of the attending anesthetist.

4

Some general comments

IMAGE ACQUISITION DIRECTION

There are certain advantages in image acquisition from bottom to top (caudad to cephalad) in some anatomical regions. Thus, in scanning the thorax, such a procedure may mean that contrast agent concentration in the central veins will be reduced from its peak by the time the upper thorax is reached, thereby reducing high-density artifacts. Breathing is also less of a problem in the upper thorax. In the liver, imaging from bottom to top increases the likelihood that the hepatic veins will be enhanced by the time they are reached. In imaging the pelvis and abdomen, beginning the scan in the pelvis at, say, 55 s after the beginning of the intravascular contrast agent infusion will give appropriate pelvic vessel and organ opacification and will mean that if imaging continues through the upper abdomen the liver will automatically be covered in the (usually) desirable portal phase.

BREATHING/BREATH-HOLDING

Scans performed in suspended inspiration are preferable to those in expiration for two reasons: patients can, of course, hold their breath longer in inspiration, and they find the 'level' easier to reproduce in inspiration for repeat acquisitions.

Some patients have difficulties with even very brief breath-holding, but the demands on them when 64-slice machines are used is minimal. Nevertheless, studies which could be taken in a single step in most patients may be broken down into two or three, perhaps overlapping, segments. It is, in any event, the case that spiral scanning and its reconstruction algorithms are robust in the face of some movement during data acquisition. For imaging of pelvic and retroperitoneal structures, respiratory excursions are quite small and breath-holding is not so important.

RADIATION EXPOSURE

CT represents the single largest medical imaging contribution to population radiation burdens, and it is incumbent upon the radiologist and radiographer to perform only appropriate examinations and to perform them in the most radiation-efficient manner compatible with obtaining the required clinical information. It is worthy of note that the higher speed and greater potential of multislice helical CT systems may lead to higher dose burdens as a result of more multiphase scanning or the application of new techniques made possible by them.

CT systems have a variety of dose-reduction systems, including one or other of: axial tube current modulation; angular tube current modulation. Such aspects should be prominent criteria in selecting a machine.

Dose burdens may be further reduced by:

(1) Planning/choosing the scanning protocol carefully – using, for example, multiple-phase scanning of the liver *only* when this is likely to give extra useful information or to deliver greater diagnostic certainty;

(2) Choosing appropriate kV and mAs.

In contrast-enhanced studies, such as CT angiography, the contrast-to-noise ratio for a fixed patient dose increases with decreasing tube voltage. As a result, to obtain a given contrast-to-noise ratio, the patient dose can be reduced by choosing lower kV settings. This effect is even more pronounced for smaller patient diameters. Studies using phantoms suggest that the required dose for the same contrast-to-noise ratio is significantly lower for lower kV values.

Not all the available machines behave in the same manner at the narrowest collimation. Only one may be used at pitch 1 while achieving the highest z-axis resolution in practice; the others need to be used at pitches of less than 1 to achieve the resolution, and this is associated with a dose increase because of overlapping 'slices'.

5

Image management

IMAGE RECONSTRUCTION

Reconstruction algorithms suggested by the manufacturer and implemented on the console software are best adopted initially. Experimentation should come later, if at all. Kernels and image filters are another subject on which it is best not to be prescriptive, and for which individual manufacturers' recommendations should be taken.

IMAGE VIEWING, REPORTING AND HARD COPY

Reviewing and reporting CT images is now undoubtedly best performed on the console, on a workstation where window levels and widths may be readily adjusted, and where multiplanar reconstructions (MPR) and other manipulations can be used to help clarify anatomical questions, or on a PACS terminal. This has been evolving as best practice for some time both as a result of the increasing amount of information (potentially numbers of images) to be processed and because of the increasing power and sophistication of workstations. The use in routine reporting of at least the axial, coronal and sagittal MPRs is strongly recommended.

Making hard copies of large numbers of images would be impractical and wasteful and, as material for reporting, would be much inferior to the original volume data set when subjected to sophisticated analysis.

Where any hard-copy images are required, as for example in a non-PACS environment, or to be taken away from the hospital to a non-PACS environment elsewhere, it is suggested that a set of image reconstructions of lower resolution (if still adequate for the purpose) or of selected images be made. The best window settings to use for hard copy depend to no small extent on the type of printing device being used, and each unit must experiment with its own equipment.

Section II:

The protocols

INTRODUCTORY REMARKS

As has been indicated earlier, the following protocols will emphasize contrast enhancement administration and timing. There will be no recommendations regarding kV, mAs, reconstruction algorithms, kernels or filters, and image hard-copying will not be discussed as it is assumed that best practice will be followed and reporting will be done on dedicated or PACS workstations. For the most part, only protocols which in themselves, or in some of their variants, involve intravascular contrast enhancement are given; dental CT and the petrous temporal bone/inner ear are included only for completion in the 'Head and neck' chapter.

The angiographic protocols have been collected in one chapter, 'CT angiography'.

A 300-mgI/ml concentration contrast agent is assumed, although some prefer higher concentrations, especially in CTA.

For the most part, 3-ml/s infusion rates are generally suggested. Some authors prefer higher rates, but the risk of extravasation increases and the gain is not great from 3 to 4 ml/s. Virtually nothing is gained above 5 ml/s.

COLLIMATION CHOICE

Multislice machines offer a wide range of different collimations. One might adopt the obvious strategy of choosing the smallest possible collimation (e.g. 0.6 mm) when high resolution is needed, and more modest collimation (e.g. 2.5 mm) when the resolution demands are not so high. However, another strategy is possible and perhaps more sensible. This is to scan everything at the smallest possible collimation (e.g. 0.6 mm) and then reconstruct, for review, more modest thickness slices, whether axial or multiplanar. This is the strategy suggested in the protocols in this book. The whole (large) data set can, if required for problem solving, be utilized on the workstation as input to one or other of the workstation tools. Of course, no one would seriously consider making hard copy of such large data sets, and one would not even wish to download to the PACS (picture archiving and communications system) such enormous amounts of data.

6

Head and neck

ROUTINE CEREBRAL CT

Indications   Suspected infarct, bleed, trauma, unconsciousness of uncertain origin, etc.

Patient position   Supine, arms down; head-rest and head-restraint recommended.

Anatomical range (topogram)   From base of skull upward.

Patient respiratory instructions   None.

Contrast enhancement   Initial non-contrast agent scan and review.

Imaging timing   —

Collimation 64×0.6 mm.

Pitch   1.

Comments:

(1)   Use of spiral rather than incremental scanning in the brain remains controversial;

(2)   Reconstruct axial sections at 6 mm above tentorium, 3 mm below; review of MPRs may be useful in some cases;

(3)   If contrast agent enhancement is indicated, use 50 ml at 3 ml/s and a 60 s delay;

(4)   For cerebral angiography, see 'CT angiography' chapter;

(5)   For detection/exclusion of fractures the data should be reconstructed a second time using a high-resolution bone kernel.

CEREBRAL PERFUSION STUDIES

Indications   Cerebral infarction, ischemia.

Patient position   Supine, arms down by side; head-rest and -restraint.

Anatomical range (See topogram)

Patient respiratory instructions   None

Contrast enhancement   50 ml at 5 ml/s.

Imaging timing   Serial scans.

Collimation   64 × 0.6 mm.

Pitch   Zero: no table feed.

Comments:

(1)   Head-rest and -restraint to prevent any head movement;

(2)   Rapid injection of compact bolus;

(3)   Unenhanced CT of brain first;

(4)   Relative cerebral volume, relative cerebral blood flow and 'time to peak' may be derived and displayed in parametric images by software of commercial machines.

ROUTINE PARANASAL SINUSES, FACIAL BONES, ORBITS

Indications   Trauma to facial bones, inflammatory disease, cysts, polyps, presurgical assessment.

Patient position   Supine, arms down, head-rest; remove dental prostheses.

Anatomical range (topogram)   Frontal sinus to alveolar ridge.

Patient respiratory instructions   None.

Contrast enhancement   None.

Imaging timing   —

Collimation   64 × 0.6 mm.

Pitch   1.

Comments:

(1) Reduction of tube current recommended since orbits are within scanned region;

(2) MPRs essential.

PARANASAL SINUSES (FOR TUMOR)

Indications   Carcinoma and other tumors, papilloma, mucocele, granulomatosis, fungal disease.

Patient position   Supine, arms down, head-rest; remove dental prostheses, etc.

Anatomical range (See topogram)

Patient respiratory instructions   None

Contrast enhancement   100 ml at 3 ml/s.

Imaging timing   40 s delay.

Collimation   64 × 0.6 mm.

Pitch   1.

Comments:

(1) Reduction of tube current recommended since orbits are within scanned region;

(2) MPRs essential;

(3) For lymph-node staging an additional neck study is necessary.

DENTAL CT

Patient position   Supine, arms down; lower shoulders as far as possible. Gantry orientation parallel to plane of teeth being imaged; place non-opaque wedge between teeth.

Anatomical range (topogram)   Entire maxilla and/or mandible.

Patient respiratory instructions   None.

Contrast enhancement   None.

Imaging timing —

Collimation   64 × 0.6 mm.

Pitch   1.

Comments:

(1)   Coronal and sagittal MPRs.

NASOPHARYNX AND OROPHARYNX

Indications   Tumor, abscess in naso- or oropharynx, salivary gland masses, skull base lesions.

Patient position   Supine, arms by sides; remove dental prostheses, etc.

Anatomical range (topogram)   Frontal sinus to superior mediastinum.

Patient respiratory instructions   Breath-hold in inspiration.

Contrast enhancement   100 ml at 3 ml/s.

Imaging timing   40 s delay.

Collimation   64 × 0.6 mm.

Pitch   1.

Comments:

(1)   MPRs useful;

(2)   Bone windows for skull base assessment.

LARYNX AND HYPOPHARYNX

Indications   Laryngeal inflammation, laryngeal tumors, laryngocele, hypopharyngeal tumor.

Patient position   Supine, arms down, remove dental prostheses, etc.

Anatomical range (topogram)   Mandible to subglottic region.

Patient respiratory instructions   Breath-hold in inspiration, then in 'e' phonation.

Contrast enhancement   100 ml at 3 ml/s.

Imaging timing   Delay 40 s – perform the two scans in quick succession.

Collimation   64 × 0.6 mm.

Pitch   1.

Comments:

(1)   Careful instruction essential to success;

(2)   'E' phonation and breath-hold scans essential when infiltration of cord suspected (T2 vs. T3 disease); shallow breathing and Valsalva maneuver sequences may also be necessary;

(3)   For nodal staging a neck study is an essential adjunct;

(4)   MPRs essential.

PETROUS TEMPORAL BONE AND INNER EAR

Indications   Post-traumatic (fracture?), cholesteatoma, otitis media, otosclerosis.

Patient position   Supine, arms down; head-rest and head-restraint recommended; remove dental prostheses, etc.

Anatomical range (topogram)   From lower end of mastoid to upper mastoid cells; avoid exposure of lens.

Patient respiratory instructions   None.

Contrast enhancement   None.

Imaging timing   —

Collimation   64 × 0.6 mm.

Pitch   1.

Comments:

(1)   Axial and coronal MPRs most useful;

(2)   The image quality with 64-slice machines obviates the need to perform a direct coronal data acquisition.

ROUTINE NECK

Indications   Cervical mass, lymphadenopathy, lymphoma staging and restaging.

Patient position   Supine, arms down by side; remove dental prostheses, etc.

Anatomical range (topogram)   Superior mediastinum to hard palate.

Patient respiratory instructions   Breath-hold in inspiration or gentle breathing (no swallowing).

Contrast enhancement   100 ml at 3 ml/s.

Imaging timing   40 s delay.

Collimation   64 × 0.6 mm.

Pitch   1.

Comments:

(1)   The fine collimation reduces dental artifacts;

(2)   MPRs useful.

7

Thorax

ROUTINE CHEST

Indications   Mediastinal and axillary adenopathy, mediastinal tumor, staging.

Patient position   Supine, arms above head.

Anatomical range (topogram)   Lung apices to below diaphragm.

Patient respiratory instructions   Breath-hold in inspiration.

Contrast enhancement   100 ml at 3 ml/s.

Imaging timing   30 s.

Collimation   64 × 0.6 mm.

Pitch   1.

Comments:

(1)   View soft tissue and lung windows;

(2)   If only lung nodules or inflammation of interest then low-dose protocol is ideal;

(3)   MPRs may be helpful.

LUNG NODULES

Indications   Lung nodules.

Patient position   Supine, arms above head.

Anatomical range (topogram)   Lung apices to below diaphragm.

Patient respiratory instructions   Breath-hold in inspiration.

Contrast enhancement   None.

Imaging timing   —

Collimation   64 × 0.6 mm.

Pitch   1.

Comments:

(1)   Breath-hold time is very brief with 64-slice machines, and within most patients' capabilities;

(2)   No contrast agent required.

COMBINATION THORAX

Indications   Examination of lungs and mediastinum.

Patient position   Supine, arms above head.

Anatomical range (topogram)   Lung apices to below diaphragm.

Patient respiratory instructions   Breath-hold in inspiration.

Contrast enhancement   100 ml at 3 ml/s.

Imaging timing   40 s.

Collimation   64 × 0.6 mm.

Pitch   1.

Comments:

(1)   Soft tissue and lung window presentations for lungs and mediastinum;

(2)   Breath-hold time is very brief with 64-slice machines, and within most patients' capabilities;

(3)   Oral barium solution may be given to improve demonstration of esophagus where desirable;

(4)   MPRs and maximum-intensity projections (MIPs) useful.

HIGH-RESOLUTION CT LUNGS

Indications   Interstitial lung disease, bronchiectasis, opportunistic infections.

Patient position   Supine, arms above the head.

Anatomical range (topogram)   Lung apices to below diaphram

Patient respiratory instructions   Breath-hold in inspiration (see comments).

Contrast enhancement   None.

Imaging timing   —

Collimation   64 × 0.6 mm.

Pitch   1.

Comments:

(1)   The isotropic high resolution offered by 64-slice machines means that spiral studies can now be performed, rather than incremental slice acquisitions;

(2)   Prone sequence, if required, may of course be more limited;

(3)   Expiration sequence, if required, may of course be more limited.

(4)   This technique may be used instead of a lower-resolution examination combined with selected high-resolution slices.

CORONARY ARTERY CALCIFICATION SCREENING

Indications   Possible coronary artery disease, atypical chest pain.

Patient position   Supine, arms elevated above head.

Anatomical range (topogram)   Bifurcation of trachea to diaphragm.

Patient respiratory instructions   Breath-hold in inspiration.

Contrast enhancement   None.

Imaging timing   —

Collimation   64 × 0.6 mm.

Pitch   1.

Comments:

(1)   Need electrocardiography (ECG) gating;

(2)   Automated scoring software needs supervision;

(3)   Check lung windows too;

(4)   For CT coronary angiography, see 'CT angiography' chapter.

8

Abdomen and pelvis

ROUTINE ABDOMEN

Indications   General screening for abdominal pathology or follow-up.

Patient position   Supine, arms elevated above head.

Anatomical range (*topogram*)   Above diaphragm to pubic symphysis.

Patient respiratory instructions   Breath-hold in inspiration.

Contrast enhancement   120 ml at 3 ml/s.

Imaging timing   65 s delay.

Collimation   64 × 0.6 mm.

Pitch   1.

Comments:

(1)   Here abdomen is taken to include pelvis;

(2)   Upper abdomen may be scanned alone (range: above diaphragm to iliac crest);

(3)   Some prefer to scan caudad to cephalad to ensure liver portal phase is established; 64-slice machines are so fast that this becomes a spurious argument.

BIPHASIC ABDOMEN/LIVER

Indications   Possible hypervascular liver metastases (e.g. carcinoid, melanoma, endocrine pancreas), hepatocellular carcinoma, adenoma and focal nodular hyperplasia.

Patient position   Supine, arms elevated above head.

Anatomical range (topogram)   From above diaphragm to iliac crest.

Patient respiratory instructions   Breath-hold in inspiration.

Contrast enhancement   120 ml at 3 ml/s.

Imaging timing   35 s and 65 s.

Collimation   64 × 0.6 mm.

Pitch   1.

Comments:

(1)   MPRs useful, especially if surgical segmental resection is planned;

(2)   MIPs useful for hepatic vascular studies.

TRIPHASIC ABDOMEN/LIVER

Indications   Characterization of lesions, e.g. hemangioma.

Patient position   Supine, arms elevated above head.

Anatomical range (topogram)   From above diaphragm to iliac crest.

Patient respiratory instructions   Breath-hold in inspiration.

Contrast enhancement   120 ml at 3 ml/s.

Imaging timing   35 s and 65 s and 120 s.

Collimation   64 × 0.6 mm.

Pitch   1.

Comments:

(1)   Hemangioma exhibits dense peripheral nodular enhancement,
filling in toward center, perhaps leaving central unfilled region.
Important characteristic is that at each phase the enhancement,
whatever its precise pattern, is the same as blood vessels.

CT ARTERIOPORTOGRAPHY

Indications   Preoperative detection of liver lesions.

Catheter placed in superior artery

Patient position   Supine, arms elevated above head.

Anatomical range (topogram)   Above diaphragm to iliac crest.

Patient respiratory instructions   Breath-hold in inspiration.

Contrast enhancement   60 ml at 3 ml/s into superior mesenteric artery.

Imaging timing   30 s and 90 s.

Collimation   64 × 0.6 mm.

Pitch   1.

Comments:

(1)   Injection may also be into splenic artery;

(2)   Two phases are necessary since there are frequently perfusion defects in the early phase;

(3)   Filling defects on a number of bases may persist in both phases; delayed CT (4–6 h) is sometimes recommended: this is based on the idea that normal hepatocytes take up a small fraction of the iodinated contrast agent, and at 4–6 h the CT number of normal liver is still sufficiently raised to render visible tumor deposits which contain abnormal or no hepatocytes;

(4)   MPRs may be useful.

CT HEPATIC ARTERIOGRAPHY

Indications   Vascular liver lesions.

Catheter placed in superior artery

Patient position   Supine, arms elevated above head.

Anatomical range (topogram)   Above diaphragm to iliac crest.

Patient respiratory instructions   Breath-hold in inspiration.

Contrast enhancement   30 ml at 2 ml/s.

Imaging timing   10 s delay.

Collimation   64 × 0.6 mm.

Pitch   1.

Comments:

(1) Technique no longer frequently used.

PANCREAS (PANCREATITIS AND FOLLOW-UP)

Indications   Pancreatitis follow-up.

Patient position   Supine, arms elevated above head.

Anatomical range (topogram)   Above diaphragm to below uncinate process.

Patient respiratory instructions   Breath-hold in inspiration.

Contrast enhancement   100 ml at 3 ml/s.

Imaging timing   65 s delay.

Collimation   64 × 0.6 mm.

Pitch   1.

Comments:

(1) Water as oral contrast agent preferred – may put patient right side down before scan is set up to fill duodenal loop.

PANCREAS (TUMOR/TUMOR STAGING)

Indications   Pancreatic tumor detection/staging.

Patient position   Supine, arms elevated above head.

Anatomical range (topogram)   First scan: above diaphragm to below uncinate process; second scan: whole upper abdomen to cover liver.

Patient respiratory instructions   Breath-hold in inspiration.

Contrast enhancement   100 ml at 3 ml/s.

Imaging timing   35 s and 65 s.

Collimation   64 × 0.6 mm.

Pitch   1.

Comments:

(1) Unenhanced upper abdominal scan first to locate pancreas;

(2)   Water as oral contrast agent preferred – may put patient right side down before scan is set up to fill duodenal loop;

(3)   Early and late arterial phases may be useful;

(4)   CT angiography essential in tumor staging.

RENAL (ROUTINE)

Indications   Follow-up of renal tumor, inflammation, infarct.

Patient position   Supine, arms elevated above head.

Anatomical range (topogram)   From mid-liver to mid-pelvis.

Patient respiratory instructions   Breath-hold in inspiration.

Contrast enhancement   100 ml at 3 ml/s.

Imaging timing   40 s.

Collimation   64 × 0.6 mm.

Pitch   1.

Comments:

(1)   MPRs useful;

(2)   If renal artery stenosis is suspected, use water as oral contrast agent and reconstruct CT angiograms;

(3)   To exclude renal vein and inferior vena cava (IVC) thrombus extend the scan up to the right atrium.

RENAL (TUMORS AND DIFFERENTIAL DIAGNOSIS)

Indications   Differential diagnosis of renal masses.

Patient position   Supine, arms elevated above head.

Anatomical range (topogram)   From mid-liver to mid-pelvis.

Patient respiratory instructions   Breath-hold in inspiration.

Contrast enhancement   100 ml at 3 ml/s.

Imaging timing   40 s (arterial or 'corticomedullary phase'), 90 s ('nephrographic phase') and 240 s ('excretory phase').

Collimation   64 × 0.6 mm.

Pitch   1.

Comments:

(1)   This triple-phase scan is useful for differential diagnosis of renal lesions, particularly tumors, but is a relatively high-dose procedure;

(2)   Significantly more lesions are detected in the 'nephrographic phase' (equal contrast in cortex and medulla) than during the 'corticomedullary phase' with its strong renal cortical enhancement and poor medullary enhancement;

(3)   The 'excretory phase' is useful for suspected renal pelvic mass;

(4)   To diagnose/exclude renal vein/IVC thrombus the second phase may be extended to the right atrium superiorly;

(5)   Renal arteriography will be obtained in first-phase scan: this may be optimized by bolus tracking with a test dose; use water as bowel contrast agent, if any.

ADRENAL GLANDS

Indications   Clinically suspected adrenal tumor, characterization of adrenal lesion.

Patient position   Supine, arms elevated above head.

Anatomical range (topogram)   Adrenals.

Patient respiratory instructions   Breath-hold in inspiration.

Contrast enhancement   120 ml at 3 ml/s.

Pre-contrast agent infusion series first

Imaging timing   50 s.

Collimation   64 × 0.6 mm.

Pitch   1.

Comments:

(1) Anxieties about precipitation by intravascular contrast agent of a hypertensive crisis in pheochromocytoma probably greatly over-played;

(2) If pheochromocytoma suspected but no adrenal lesion, extend coverage to include aortic bifurcation and urinary bladder;

(3) Characterization of lesions is to some extent possible: CT number < 10 on unenhanced scan suggests adenoma; or can take measure of 'wash-out'.

COMBINATION SCANS: NECK, THORACIC, ABDOMINOPELVIC

In the past, some thought had to be given to how best to cover multiple areas. Where was a breath-hold essential and where not? Could the whole range in question reasonably be covered on a single breath-hold or should separate scans with intervals be done? Would contrast enhancement be sufficient throughout the scan in all regions? Now the 64-slice machines are so fast that all regions can be taken in one scan on a single breath-hold, and, assuming that timing is correct in the first place, there is no likelihood that contrast enhancement in one body part covered is good and in another, is not good.

CT PNEUMOCOLON

Indications   Detection of large bowel tumors/polyps.

Patient position   Supine, arms elevated above head.

Anatomical range (topogram)   Above diaphragm to pubic symphysis.

Patient respiratory instructions   Breath-hold in inspiration.

Contrast enhancement   120 ml at 3 ml/s.

Imaging timing   65 s delay.

Collimation   64 × 0.6 mm.

Pitch   1.

Comments:

(1)   Scan caudad to cephalad;

(2)   Check sufficient air insufflation using scanogram;

(3)   May need to repeat with patient prone;

(4)   MPRs useful; virtual colonoscopy/'flythrough' desirable;

(5)   Liver is automatically included in the appropriate portal phase.

CT ENTEROCLYSIS

Indications   Evaluation of small bowel – inflammatory processes, infiltration, primary and metastatic disease.

Patient position   Supine, arms elevated above head.

Anatomical range (topogram)   Above diaphragm to pubic symphysis.

Patient respiratory instructions   Breath-hold in inspiration.

Oral contrast agent   Methylcellulose via nasogastric tube.

Contrast enhancement   120 ml at 3 ml/s.

Imaging timing   60 s delay.

Collimation   64 × 0.6 mm.

Pitch   1.

Comments:

(1)   MPRs helpful.

TRAUMA

Indications   To exclude or detect soft-tissue or bony injuries following trauma.

Patient position   Supine, arms elevated above head.

Anatomical range (topogram)   Head to toe.

Patient respiratory instructions   None if patient unable to cooperate.

Contrast enhancement   Ideally 120 ml at 3 ml/s, but may be abandoned in cases needing very urgent assessment.

Imaging timing　65 s delay (if contrast agent given).

Collimation　64 × 0.6 mm.

Pitch　1.5.

Comments:

(1)　Can be done in little over 15 s with a rotation time of 0.375 s;

(2)　May need to tailor examination to particular regions of high suspicion;

(3)　MPRs useful;

(4)　Bone and soft-tissue window reviews;

(5)　May need to do an arteriogram.

9

CT angiography

CEREBRAL ANGIOGRAPHY

Indications   Intracranial aneurysm, arteriovenous malformation, arterial thrombosis.

Patient position   Supine, arms by sides; head-rest and head-restraint recommended; remove dental prostheses, etc.

Anatomical range (topogram)   Skull base to vertex.

Patient respiratory instructions   None.

Contrast enhancement   100 ml at 3 ml/s.

Imaging timing   Typically 40 s delay, but use bolus-timing software.

Collimation   64 × 0.6 mm.

Pitch   1.

Comments:

(1)   MPRs, MIPs and volume-rendering technique (VRT) all useful;

(2)   Perform routine head protocol first.

VENOUS SINUS ANGIOGRAPHY

Indications   Suspected thrombosis of venous sinuses or of large cerebral veins.

Patient position   Supine, arms by sides; remove dental prostheses, etc.

Anatomical range (topogram)   Skull base to vertex.

Patient respiratory instructions   None.

Contrast enhancement   100 ml at 3 ml/s.

Imaging timing   100 s.

Collimation   64 × 0.6 mm.

Pitch   1.

Comments:

(1)   A routine head protocol should be carried out first;

(2)   MPRs and MIPs essential;

(3)   This technique is probably not capable of detecting or excluding a cavernous sinus or cephalic vein thrombosis.

CAROTID ANGIOGRAPHY

Indications   Suspected stenosis, occlusion or dissection of carotid artery or branches.

Patient position   Supine, arms by sides; remove dental prostheses, etc.

Anatomical range (topogram)   Sternal notch to sella.

Patient respiratory instructions   Breath-hold in inspiration.

Contrast enhancement   100 ml at 3 ml/s.

Imaging timing   Use bolus timing.

Collimation   64 × 0.6 mm.

Pitch   1.

Comments:

(1)   Optimize timing using timing software;

(2)   MPRs, MIPs and VRT may all be useful in image analysis.

PULMONARY ANGIOGRAPHY

Indications   Detection/exclusion of pulmonary embolus.

Patient position   Supine, arms elevated above head.

Anatomical range (topogram)   From aortic arch though central hilar regions.

Patient respiratory instructions   Breath-hold in inspiration.

Contrast enhancement   100 ml at 3 ml/s.

Imaging timing   Typically 20 s delay, but determine by bolus tracking.

Collimation   64 × 0.6 mm.

Pitch   1.

Comments:

(1)   MPRs and MIPs may both be helpful;

(2)   Examine right heart as source of embolus.

CORONARY ARTERIOGRAPHY

Indications   Suspected coronary artery disease.

Patient position   Supine, arms elevated above head.

Anatomical range (topogram)   Above tracheal bifurcation to below diaphragm.

Patient respiratory instructions   Breath-hold in inspiration.

Contrast enhancement   40 ml at 4 ml/s followed by 80 ml at 2 ml/s (variable-rate injector).

Imaging timing   Commence 10 s after start of second phase of infusion.

Collimation   64 × 0.6 mm.

Rotation time   0.33 s preferred if available.

Pitch   1.

Comments:

(1)   ECG gating is essential;

(2)   If cardiac rate is very fast, beta-blockade should be considered;

(3)   Use test bolus to establish timing;

(4)   MIPs and VRT essential;

(5)   Quality of non-invasive CT coronary arteriography with 64-slice machines is now very close to that of catheter angiography.

CORONARY ARTERY BYPASS GRAFT ASSESSMENT

Indications   Follow-up after coronary artery bypass surgery.

Patient position   Supine, arms elevated above head.

Anatomical range (topogram)   Aortic arch to below diaphragm.

Patient respiratory instructions   Breath-hold in inspiration.

Contrast enhancement   40 ml at 4 ml/s followed by 80 ml at 2 ml/s (variable-rate injector).

Imaging timing   Commence 10 s after start of second phase of infusion.

Collimation 64×0.6 mm.

Rotation time   0.33 s preferred if available.

Pitch   1.

Comments:

(1)   Test bolus essential to establish timing;

(2)   Retrospective or prospective ECG gating essential;

(3)   MIPs and VRT essential;

(4)   Other planes essential – e.g. 45° oblique parallel to mainstem;

(5)   Cardiac rate ideally less than 70/s – may consider beta-blockade.

AORTOGRAPHY

Thoracic aortography

Indications   Detection/exclusion of aortic aneurysm, dissection, bleeding or thrombosis of the ascending aorta, aortic arch or descending thoracic aorta.

Patient position   Supine, arms extended above head.

Anatomical range (topogram)   Lung apices to below diaphragm.

Patient respiratory instructions   Breath-hold in inspiration.

Contrast enhancement   120 ml at 3 ml/s.

Imaging timing   20 s delay or use bolus-timing technique.

Collimation   64 × 0.6 mm.

Pitch   1.

Comments:

(1)   Caudad to cephalad scanning is desirable – may reduce high-contrast agent concentration venous inflow artifact and, if breath-holding is a problem, the greater-excursion-of-movement lower parts are scanned first;

(2)   MPRs and MIPs essential;

(3)   A bolus-timing technique is useful.

Abdominal aortography

Indications   Detection/exclusion of aortic aneurysm, dissection, retroperitoneal bleeding or thrombosis of the descending aorta.

Patient position   Supine, arms extended above head.

Anatomical range (topogram)   Above diaphragm to symphysis pubis.

Patient respiratory instructions   Breath-hold in inspiration.

Contrast enhancement   120 ml at 3 ml/s.

Imaging timing   20 s delay or use bolus-timing technique.

Collimation   64 × 0.6 mm.

Pitch   1.

Comments:

(1)   MPRs and MIPs essential;

(2)   A bolus-timing technique is useful;

(3)   With a 64-slice machine, coverage of thoracic and abdominal aorta in one sweep in a single breath-hold is easily achieved.

VISCERAL ANGIOGRAPHY

Indications   Assessment of abdominovisceral arterial disease, disease staging (vascular involvement) and venography (e.g. portography).

All visceral arteriography may be achieved using the abdominal aorta protocol above. The whole abdomen may be examined if appropriate or a region of interest, e.g. for renal arteriography.

Perform a second scan for the venous phase 20 s later.

Comments:

(1)   A bolus-timing technique is useful;

(2)   MPRs and MIPs essential.

PERIPHERAL ANGIOGRAPHY

Indications   Peripheral vascular disease.

Patient position   Supine, arms elevated above head.

Anatomical range (topogram)   Above renal arteries to ankles.

Patient respiratory instructions   None

Contrast enhancement   120 ml at 3 ml/s.

Imaging timing   25–30 s but timing method recommended.

Collimation   64 × 0.6 mm.

Pitch   1.

Comments:

(1)   MIPs, MPRs and VRT recommended;

(2)   A unilateral stenosis may pose timing problems;

(3)   See discussion of 'CT angiography' in Section 1 for theoretical considerations.

Bibliography

Bae TB, Heiken JP, Brink JA. Aortic and hepatic peak enhancement at CT: effect of contrast medium injection rate: pharmacokinetic analysis and experimental porcine model. Radiology 1998; 206: 455–64

Bae KT, Heiken JP, Brink JA. Aortic and hepatic contrast medium enhancement at CT Part I: Prediction with a computer model. Radiology 1998; 207: 647–55

Bae KT, Heiken JP, Brink JA. Aortic and hepatic contrast medium enhancement at CT Part II: Effect of reduced cardiac output in a porcine model. Radiology 1998; 207: 657–62

Blomley MJK, Coulden R, Dawson P, et al. Liver perfusion studies with ultrafast CT. J Comput Assist Tomogr 1995; 19: 424–33

Blomley MJK, Coulden R, Kormano M, et al. Splenic blood flow, evaluation with CT. Acad Radiol 1997; 4: 13–20

Blomley MJK, Dawson P. Contrast bolus dynamic CT for the measurement of solid organ perfusion. Invest Radiol 1993; 28: 572–7

Blomley MJK, Dawson P. The quantification of renal function with computerised tomography. Br J Radiol 1996; 69: 989–95

Blomley MJK, Dawson P. Bolus dynamics: theoretical and experimental aspects. Br J Radiol 1997; 70: 351–9

Blomley MJK, Harvey CJ, Jager RG, et al. Functional renal perfusion imaging with colour mapping: is it a useful adjunct to spiral CT in the assessment of abdominal aortic aneurysm? Eur J Radiol 1999; 30: 214–20

Dawson P. Factors determining tumour contrast enhancement–time curves. Acad Radiol 1998; 5: S228–30

Dawson P. Dynamic contrast-enhanced functional imaging with multislice CT. Acad Radiol 2002; 9 (Suppl 2): S368–S376

Dawson P. Emerging issues in multidetector computed tomography imaging. J Comput Assist Tomogr 2003; 27 (Suppl 1): S2

Dawson P, Blomley MJK. Contrast agent pharmacokinetics revisited. I. Reformulation. Acad Radiol 1995; 3: S261–3

Dawson P, Blomley MJK. Contrast agent pharmacokinetics revisited. II. Computer aided analysis. Acad Radiol 1995; 3: S264–7

Dawson P, Blomley MJK. Contrast media as extracellular fluid space markers; adaptation of the central volume theorem. Br J Radiol 1996; 69: 717–22

Dawson P, Blomley MJK. The value of mathematical modelling in the design of protocols in clinical CT. Eur J Radiol 2002; 41: 222–36

Dawson P, Cosgrove DO. A Textbook of Contrast Enhancing Agents. London: Martin Dunitz, 2000

Dawson P, Lees WR. Multi-slice spiral CT. Clin Radiol 2001; 56: 302–9

Dawson P, Miles KA, Blomley MJK. Functional CT. Oxford: ISIS Medical Media Ltd, 1997

Dawson P, Morgan J. On the meaning and significance of the equilibrium point in clinical CT. Br J Radiol 1999; 172: 438–42

Dawson P, Peters AM. Dynamic bolus contrast CT of the kidney. A functional study. Invest Radiol 1993; 18: 1039–42

Dawson P, Peters AM. Functional imaging in CT. The use of contrast enhanced CT for the study of renal function and physiology. Invest Radiol 1993; 28: 579–84

Dawson P, Peters AM. What is the nephrogram? Br J Radiol 1993; 67: 21–5

Dawson P, Peters AM. Renal function and the excretion of contrast agent. Br J Radiol 1996; 69: 567–9

Harvey C, Dooher A, Morgan J, et al. Imaging of tumour therapy responses by dynamic CT. Eur J Radiol 1999; 30: 221–6

Harvey C, Blomley MJ, Dawson P. Functional CT imaging of the acute hyperaemic response to radiation therapy of the prostate gland: early experience. J Comput Assist Tomogr 2001; 25: 43–9

Harvey C, Morgan J, Blomley M, et al. Tumour responses to radiation therapy: use of dynamic contrast material-enhanced CT to monitor functional and anatomical indices. Acad Radiol 2002; 9 (Suppl 1): S215–19

Krause W. Application of pharmacokinetics to computed tomography. Injection rates and schemes: mono-, bi-, or multiphasic. Invest Radiol 1996; 31: 91–100

Index

Protocol descriptions have a standard format describing: indications, patient position, anatomical range, patient respiratory instructions, contrast enhancement, imaging timing, collimation, pitch and comments. Apart from 'indications' these have not been indexed separately. Protocols and techniques have page references in **bold**.

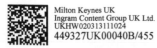

Milton Keynes UK
Ingram Content Group UK Ltd.
UKHW020313111024
449327UK00040B/455